I0493824

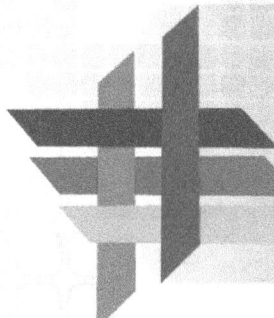

Data Security and Confidentiality Guidelines

for HIV, Viral Hepatitis, Sexually Transmitted Disease, and Tuberculosis Programs:

Standards to Facilitate Sharing and Use of Surveillance Data for Public Health Action

National Center for HIV/AIDS, Viral Hepatitis, STD, and TB Prevention

CDC

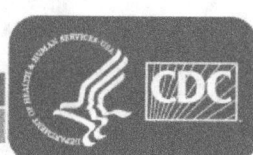

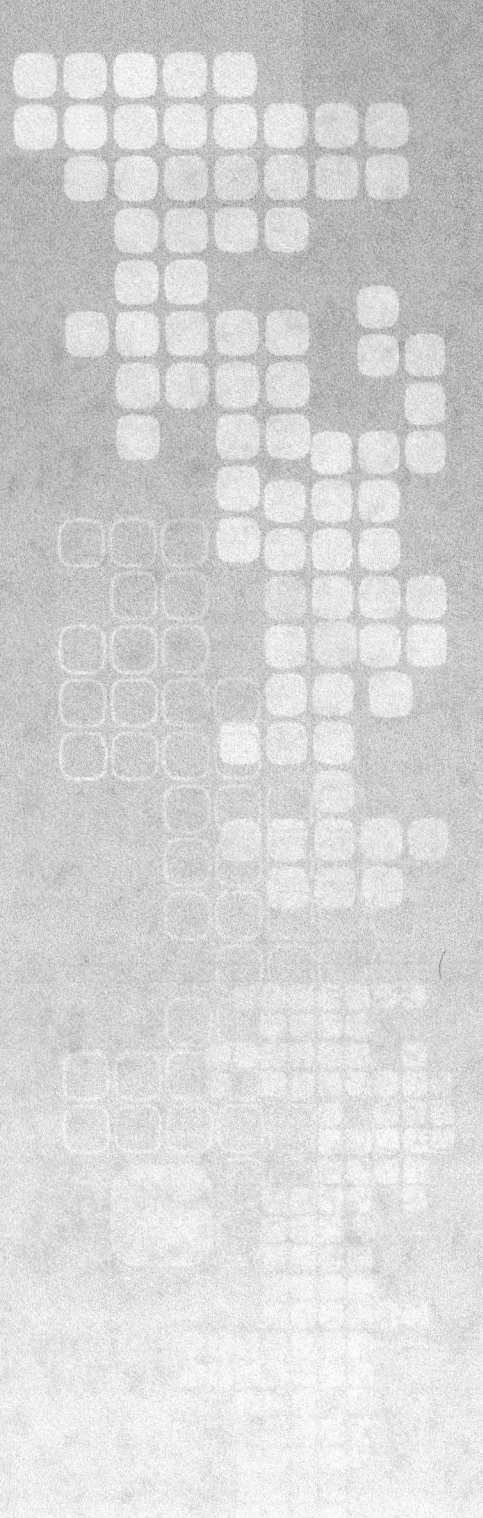

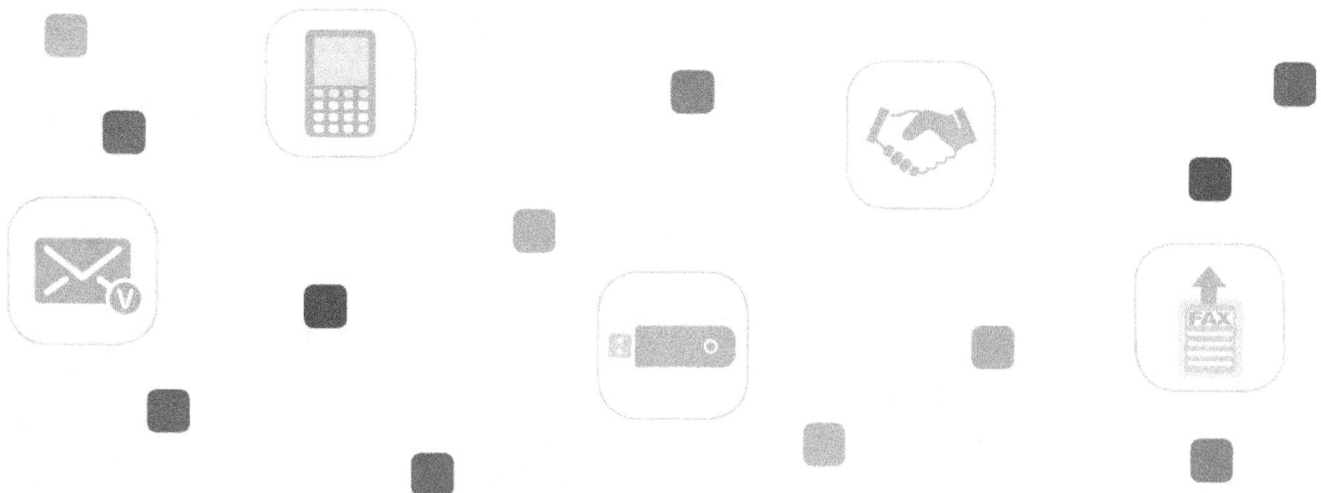

Data Security and Confidentiality Guidelines

for HIV, Viral Hepatitis, Sexually Transmitted Disease, and Tuberculosis Programs:

Standards to Facilitate Sharing and Use of Surveillance Data for Public Health Action

Suggested Citation: Centers for Disease Control and Prevention. Data Security and
Confidentiality Guidelines for HIV, Viral Hepatitis, Sexually Transmitted Disease, and Tuberculosis Programs:
Standards to Facilitate Sharing and Use of Surveillance Data for Public Health Action.
Atlanta (GA): U.S. Department of Health and Human Services, Centers for Disease Control and Prevention; 2011

This report was prepared by

**Security and Confidentiality Guidelines Subgroup
of CDC's NCHHSTP Surveillance Work Group:**

Patricia Sweeney, Sam Costa;
Division of HIV/AIDS Prevention

Hillard Weinstock , Patrick Harris, Nicholas Gaffga;
Division of STD Prevention

Kashif Iqbal;
Division of Viral Hepatitis

Lilia Manangan, Suzanne Marks;
Division of TB Elimination

Gustavo Aquino;
Office of the Director, NCHHSTP

Table of Contents

I. Executive Summary

A goal of CDC's National Center for HIV/AIDS, Viral Hepatitis, STD, and TB Prevention (NCHHSTP) is to strengthen collaborative work across disease areas and integrate services that are provided by state and local programs* for prevention of HIV/AIDS, viral hepatitis, other sexually transmitted diseases (STDs), and tuberculosis (TB). A major barrier to achieving this goal is the lack of standardized data security and confidentiality procedures, which has often been cited as an obstacle for programs seeking to maximize use of data for public health action and provide integrated and comprehensive services.

Maintaining confidentiality and security of public health data is a priority across all public health programs. However, policies vary and although disease-specific standards exist for CDC-funded HIV programs, similarly comprehensive CDC standards are lacking for viral hepatitis, STD, and TB prevention programs. Successful implementation of common data protections in state and local health departments with integrated programs suggest implementation of common data security and confidentiality policies is both reasonable and feasible. These programs have benefited from enhanced successful collaborations citing increased completeness of key data elements, collaborative analyses, and gains in program efficiencies as important benefits. Despite the potential benefits, however, policies have not been consistently implemented and the absence of common standards is frequently cited as impeding data sharing and use. Adoption of common practices for securing and protecting data will provide a critical foundation and be increasingly important for ensuring the appropriate sharing and use of data as programs begin to modify policies and increasingly use data for public health action.

This document recommends standards for all NCHHSTP programs that, when adopted, will facilitate the secure collection, storage, and use of data while maintaining confidentiality. Designed to support the most desirable practices for enabling secure use of surveillance data for public health action and ensuring implementation of comprehensive evidence-based prevention services, the standards are based on 10 guiding principles that provide the foundation for the collection, storage, and use of these public health data. They address five areas: program policies and responsibilities, data collection and use, data sharing and release, physical security, and electronic data security. Intended for use by state and local health department disease programs to inform the development of policies and procedures, the standards are intentionally broad to allow for differences in public health activities and response across disease programs.

The standards, and the guiding principles from which they are derived, are meant to serve as the foundation for more detailed policy development by programs and as a basis for determining if and where improvements are needed. The process includes seven main steps: designating an overall responsible party; performing a standards-based initial assessment of data security and confidentiality protections; developing and maintaining written data security policies and procedures based on assessment findings; developing and implementing training; developing data-sharing plans or agreements as needed; certification of adherence to standards; and

*State and local is inclusive of state, tribal, local and territorial health departments and agencies.

performing periodic reviews of policies and procedures. NCHHSTP-funded programs will also be required to verify their adherence to the standards through submission of certification statements. CDC will work with state and local health departments to monitor the implementation of the guidelines and evaluate their impact on securing data, facilitating data use, and increasing program effectiveness.

This document reflects the combined efforts of NCHHSTP's Surveillance Workgroup members, composed of surveillance leaders from NCHHSTP's Division of HIV/AIDS Prevention (DHAP), Division of Viral Hepatitis (DVH), Division of STD Prevention (DSTDP), and Division of TB Elimination (DTBE). The work was informed by consultation with state and local public health leaders and public health organizations representing HIV, viral hepatitis, STD and TB disease disciplines (see Acknowledgements section). The document supersedes previously published security and confidentiality guidelines for HIV surveillance and establishes data security and confidentiality standards for viral hepatitis, STD, and TB. Establishment of these standards that apply to all surveillance activities in all of the Center's divisions will facilitate collaboration and service integration among NCHHSTP-funded programs with minimal risk of inappropriate release of confidential, identifiable surveillance data or misuse of those data in pursuit of legitimate public health purposes.

II. Introduction

The true value of surveillance is measured by its impact on public health action and practice.[1] Public health agencies at all levels have broad authority to collect, store, and use personal health information to identify, report, and control health threats and to plan, implement, and evaluate public health programs and services. The public trusts that any personal or confidential information collected as part of public health activities will be held securely and confidentially and will be used for legitimate public health purposes. Although protections exist through various laws, policies and procedures, these protections vary across jurisdictions[2-4] and sometimes even within public health organizations.[5]

A goal of CDC's National Center for HIV/AIDS, Viral Hepatitis, STD, and TB Prevention (NCHHSTP) is to strengthen collaborative work across disease areas and integrate services that are provided by programs for prevention of HIV/AIDS, viral hepatitis, other sexually transmitted diseases (STDs), and tuberculosis (TB).[6] A major barrier to achieving this goal is the lack of standardized data security and confidentiality procedures, which has often been cited as an obstacle for programs seeking to maximize use of data for public health action and provide integrated and comprehensive services.[7] Although disease-specific standards exist for CDC-funded HIV programs,[8,9] similarly comprehensive CDC standards are lacking for viral hepatitis, STD, and TB prevention programs.

CDC established data security and confidentiality guidelines for CDC-funded HIV surveillance programs in state and local* health departments in 1998[8] and updated the guidelines in 2006.[9] The guidelines emphasize the protection of surveillance data and prohibit HIV surveillance programs from sharing data with programs that lack equivalent data security and confidentiality protections. These restrictions on data sharing had the unintended consequence of inhibiting the ability of some local health departments to link clients to appropriate treatment and prevention services.[7,10]

In 2008, CDC published updated recommendations for programs providing partner services for HIV, syphilis, gonorrhea, and chlamydial infections. The document includes recommendations related to record keeping, data collection, data management, and data security that were based on previously published HIV surveillance guidelines.[11] The partner services recommendations encourage data linkage and sharing between public health service-provision prevention programs and disease-reporting surveillance systems. The recommendations suggest that sharing of individual-level surveillance data can help facilitate the timely provision of partner services but also underscore the need for well-defined security and confidentiality policies and procedures. Despite the potential benefits, however, these have not been consistently implemented.

In addition, CDC cooperative agreements with TB programs require that policies and procedures must be in place to protect the confidentiality of all TB surveillance case reports and files. TB programs should also collaborate with HIV/AIDS programs to conduct at least annual TB and AIDS registry matches to ensure completeness of reporting of HIV and TB coinfected patients to both surveillance systems. However, this collaboration has been hampered by perceived differences in policies and procedures to protect HIV test results.

This document does not specify details of how, what or when data should be shared but rather establishes standards of data protection across programs that should be in place. Intended for use by state and local health department disease programs to inform the development of policies and procedures, the standards are intentionally broad to allow for necessary differences in public health activities and response across disease programs. The extent to which data are used for public health interventions and follow-up with individuals, and to which health department programs interact or share data with reporting physicians and health providers, will vary according to established program practices.

This document reflects the combined efforts of NCHHSTP's Surveillance Workgroup members, composed of surveillance leaders from NCHHSTP's Division of HIV/AIDS Prevention (DHAP), Division of Viral Hepatitis (DVH), Division of STD Prevention (DSTDP), and Division of TB Elimination (DTBE). The document supersedes previously published guidelines for HIV surveillance and partner services and establishes up-to-date data security and confidentiality standards of viral hepatitis, STD, and TB.

---

*State and local is inclusive of state, tribal, local and territorial health departments and agencies.

Key Definitions Used in this Document

Data sharing: Granting certain individuals or organizations access to data that contain personally identifiable information with the understanding that personally identifiable or potentially identifiable data cannot be re-released further unless a special data-sharing agreement governs the use and re-release of the data and is agreed upon by the receiving program and the data provider(s).

Data-sharing agreement: Mechanism by which a data requestor and data provider can define the terms of data access that can be granted to requestors.

Data release: Dissemination of data either in a public-use file or as a result of an ad hoc request which results in the data steward no longer controlling the use of the data. Data may be released in a variety of formats including, but not limited to, tables, microdata (person records), or online query systems.

Data dissemination: Any mechanism by which data are made available to users. Includes mechanisms whereby data are released to users as well as mechanisms whereby data are made available without being released.

Personally identifiable information: As defined by National Institute of Standards and Technology Special Publication 800-34, Guide To Protecting The Confidentiality of Personally Identifiable Information: "Any information about an individual maintained by an agency, including (1) any information that can be used to distinguish or trace an individual's identity, such as name, social security number, date and place of birth, mother's maiden name, or biometric records; and (2) any other information that is linked or linkable to an individual, such as medical, educational, financial, and employment information."[12]

Adapted from: CDC/ATSDR data release guidelines and procedures for re-release of state-provided data.[4] See glossary in Appendix A for additional definitions of terms used in this document.

III. About this Document

This document recommends standards for data security, confidentiality, and use across surveillance and program areas for HIV, viral hepatitis, STD, and TB prevention in state and local health jurisdictions. The standards support the most desirable practices for enabling secure use of data and ensuring comprehensive preventive services while being broad enough to allow for differences in public health activities by disease program. The standards address five areas: program policies and responsibilities, data collection and use, data sharing and release, physical security, and electronic data security.

The standards are based on 10 guiding principles that provide the foundation for the collection, storage, and use of surveillance data for public health action. The guiding principles are derived from existing CDC policies and guidelines, model and existing legislation, and from related work, including current security and confidentiality principles for NCHHSTP's HIV surveillance programs and practical application of ethics in public health surveillance.[8,9,11,13-20] Similar principles have been proposed as part of a national strategy[21] consistent with public health values[22,23] to ensure the privacy and security of public health data at all levels.

The standards are intended to apply to public health programs funded by NCHHSTP (including those of state and local health departments and their contractors) that are responsible for collecting, storing, and using surveillance data and to any entities with which these programs share data. The standards address the use of both identifiable (i.e., personally identifiable information [PII]) and nonidentifiable data and may include: data used for epidemiologic investigations; data used to link patients with partner services, appropriate treatment, interventions, and other health services; and data used for case management and program evaluation. Because the use of identifiable data requires a higher level of protection than the use of nonidentifiable data, the document includes specific standards for the sharing of identifiable data. Key definitions for data sharing, data release, data release agreement, data dissemination, and personally identifiable information are highlighted in the box above and additional terms are provided in the Glossary (Appendix A).

IV. Using this Document

Active data stewardship involves developing proactive policies, procedures, and training to ensure that public health data are collected, stored, and used appropriately. To that end, policies related to the security and sharing of data should be reviewed regularly and changed as needed. The data standards and the guiding principles from which they are derived are meant to serve as the foundation for more detailed policy development by programs and as a basis for determining if and where improvements are needed. Key components of data security and confidentiality, sharing, and use policy development are outlined below.

Overall Responsible Party (ORP)—A high-ranking official should be identified to accept overall responsibility for implementing and enforcing data security, confidentiality and sharing standards. This official should have the authority to make decisions about program operations that might affect programs authorizing, accessing or using the data, and should serve as the contact for public health professionals regarding security and confidentiality policies and practices. If the required span of control is not under a single person's purview, several persons can serve in the capacity of ORP as an ORP panel.

Initial Assessment of Data Security and Confidentiality Protections—This document is intended to serve as a planning resource for use by state and local public health programs to develop or upgrade their data security and confidentiality policies and procedures. An initial assessment will be particularly useful for state and local public health programs that currently lack data security and confidentiality policies and procedures.

A team led by the ORP should conduct an initial assessment of current data security and confidentiality protections. The team should include:

- Program managers, directors, or equivalent leaders from participating programs

- Other representatives of participating programs who may provide insight on access requirements and procedures for certain jobs or duties (e.g., surveillance staff, DIS data managers)

- Staff members with technical expertise in data security

Information technology (IT) staff should be involved at an early stage to ensure that they understand the data security and confidentiality standards and are fully engaged in the overall process. This involvement is critical as areas move to more centralized IT services and, in some cases, outsourced IT services.

The initial assessment should include the following steps:

- Identify key individuals and designate an ORP or ORP panel

- Review current security and confidentiality-related materials (e.g., written policies, procedures)

- Review relevant state and local laws that might affect data security and confidentiality policies

- Identify any policies or procedures that are either sources of data security weaknesses or barriers to information sharing and consult standard operating procedures (SOPs) from other programs that might be useful sources of ideas or suggestions for procedural changes

- Review any history of data security breaches or near-breaches, and associated lessons learned

- Assess physical security and define the secure area

- Assess electronic security protections and methods of electronic data transfer and storage

- Assess factors related to security of information in the field

- Assess training needs

Sample checklists for conducting initial and comprehensive assessments are provided in Appendix B.

Data Security and Confidentiality Policies and Procedures—Programs required by NCHHSTP to meet these guidelines are responsible for developing and maintaining written, program-specific data security and confidentiality policies and standard operating procedures, based on these guidelines, the assessment findings and in the context of state and local laws. Legislative and regulatory barriers to these standards should be addressed. State health department programs should work collaboratively with local health departments and public health partners involved in surveillance and prevention-related activities to maintain equivalent standards to the extent possible. State programs that subcontract directly with local health department programs may include compliance with these guidelines in their contractual arrangements. Local health departments that share data with state health departments should share data using the secure methods outlined in this document. NCHHSTP-funded programs may provide assistance to private providers and laboratories in implementing secure methods for reporting case data. Providers and laboratories should be encouraged to establish policies and procedures and regular training on data security and confidentiality, according to these standards.

When public health data are collected or used as part of federally funded research, they are also subject to the federal policy for the protection of human subjects as described in the Code of Federal Regulations, Title 45, Part 46.[24]

Training—Staff members authorized to access and use public health data are responsible for adhering to their programs' data security and confidentiality policies and procedures and should receive ongoing training on an annual basis on the appropriate collection, storage, use, and dissemination of data as defined by these policies.

Data-Sharing Plans—Shared data facilitates identification of populations at risk for multiple infections and the design and implementation of programs that comprehensively address identified needs. A written plan can serve as a starting point for discussions about data sharing between or among public health programs. A data-sharing plan should include:

- Intent and scope of data sharing

- Potential benefits (including projected efficiencies) and risks of sharing, benefits and risks of not sharing, and methods to monitor these benefits and risks

- Methods that will be used to share data and roles and responsibilities of staff involved

- Minimum data elements needed to achieve the objective(s), including need for PII

- Steps that will be taken to ensure the confidentiality and security of shared data

- Provisions for physical and electronic security

- How shared data will be used, analyzed, published, released, and retained/destroyed

- Confidentiality agreements

- Knowledge and training requirements including annual training for staff who have access to PII and non-PII data

Although a written plan might not seem necessary between programs in the same health department or in integrated programs, having a plan in writing can help in resolving any conflicts. A more formal agreement, such as a data-sharing agreement or Memorandum of Understanding (MOU) may be required in certain circumstances (e.g., sharing outside the health department or with another public health organization). Programs can consult legal experts in their organizations to determine the need for a formal agreement.

Appendix C includes an example of one method of data sharing to improve program efficiencies and effectiveness.

Certification—Programs are required to self-certify their adherence to the standards for ensuring the security, confidentiality, and appropriate use of the data they collect, store, and share. The certification statement should:

- Identify one or more persons as the ORP for ensuring adherence to the standards

- Attest to adherence to all standards, or explain any lapses

- If lapses, describe steps to meet the standards in the future

- Describe policies and procedures instituted to ensure continued adherence to the standards

NCHHSTP will describe the certification process in applicable program announcements. NCHHSTP will conduct periodic reviews of the data security, confidentiality and sharing procedures of grant recipients during routine site visits and provide technical assistance as needed.

A suggested format for a certification statement is provided in Appendix D.

Periodic and Ongoing Reviews and Assessments—Programs should review their data security, confidentiality, and sharing policies and procedures at least annually or sooner if improved technologies or legislative/regulatory changes occur and revise as necessary. In addition, they should periodically assess whether other changes in personnel, programs, organizations, or priorities require changes in policies and procedures. For example, changes in federal standards for encryption could affect existing policies and procedures and require software updates or other revisions.

Programs should also review their data-sharing plans or agreements periodically in light of improved technologies and revise as necessary. Tracking the security and confidentiality training of staff members authorized to access data, including documenting and storing their signed confidentiality agreements, should also be part of ongoing assessment activities.

V. Benefits, Risks, and Costs of Sharing Data and Maintaining Security and Confidentiality

There is a balance that must be maintained between protecting the individual and the public from disease and protecting individuals' confidentiality and right to privacy. Both are vital to enhancing the public's health and maintaining the public's trust. Programs that have and follow consistent guidelines for the collection, storage, and use of HIV, viral hepatitis, STD, and TB data may reassure individuals, and the public, that sharing data for public health action will not compromise confidentiality.

Adherence to harmonized standards for data security across programs will enhance the ability to share data without compromising confidentiality. As programs consider how best to meet these standards, it is helpful to consider the benefits, risks, and costs. The public health benefits of sharing data among HIV, viral hepatitis, STD, and TB programs include the following:

- Early case detection and accurate and timely reporting of diseases

- Improved efficiencies in use of human and financial resources to achieve program objectives

- Improved projections of human and financial resources for disease programs and specific projects

- Improved opportunities to inform providers and patients about standards of care and needs for additional care

- Enhanced quality of surveillance data across programs

- Improved documentation and reporting of co-morbidities, leading to better patient management and partner services

- Better understanding of patients' health status to ensure comprehensive care and avoid redundant services and missed opportunities for prevention

- Increased understanding of how epidemics interact synergistically (syndemics), geographically, within population subgroups, or within groups engaging in specified high-risk behaviors

- Identification of specific populations that need outreach with consistent messages and targeted testing and service provision

Although data sharing has many benefits, there are also some risks. Despite the public health community's excellent track record in managing sensitive data, security breaches can occur. Harmonized data security and confidentiality standards among programs, and a commitment to enforcing them, can, however, minimize these risks. Breaches involving electronic data with identifiable information (e.g., human error resulting in reports going to the wrong patient or provider or databases being stolen or accessed illegally) might cause greater harm because more information about more individuals is released. Therefore, procedures for electronic data security must be developed. However, there are also some risks to not sharing data. Individuals might not receive prevention services, clients might not receive appropriate treatment, clients might not receive treatment at all, and disease transmission might increase.

Costs associated with improvements in data security can be a barrier to data sharing. To facilitate data sharing, hardware and software systems need to be compatible. Electronic transfer of data needs to be performed securely. Storage of data needs to be secure and remain confidential at all levels. Additional computer programming support may be required to facilitate secure data sharing across programs, conduct data matches, meet systems requirements, and de-duplicate data.

VI. Guiding Principles for Data Collection, Storage, Sharing, and Use to Ensure Security and Confidentiality

The 10 principles below are intended to guide NCHHSTP-funded programs in developing data security and confidentiality policies. The principles should guide the collection, storage, and use of data for legitimate public health purposes. Legitimate public health purposes can be defined as a population-based activity or individual effort aimed primarily at the prevention of injury, disease, or premature mortality. This term also refers to the promotion of health in the community, including 1) assessing the health needs and status of the community through public health surveillance and epidemiologic research; 2) developing public health policy; and 3) responding to public health needs and emergencies. Public health purposes can include analysis and evaluation of conditions of public health importance and evaluation of public health programs. The principles also underpin the data security standards defined in the following section.

TEN GUIDING PRINCIPLES FOR DATA COLLECTION, STORAGE, SHARING, AND USE TO ENSURE SECURITY AND CONFIDENTIALITY

1. Public health data should be acquired, used, disclosed, and stored for legitimate public health purposes.

2. Programs should collect the minimum amount of personally identifiable information necessary to conduct public health activities.

3. Programs should have strong policies to protect the privacy and security of personally identifiable data.

4. Data collection and use policies should reflect respect for the rights of individuals and community groups and minimize undue burden.

5. Programs should have policies and procedures to ensure the quality of any data they collect or use.

6. Programs have the obligation to use and disseminate summary data to relevant stakeholders in a timely manner.

7. Programs should share data for legitimate public health purposes and may establish data-use agreements to facilitate sharing data in a timely manner.

8. Public health data should be maintained in a secure environment and transmitted through secure methods.

9. Minimize the number of persons and entities granted access to identifiable data.

10. Program officials should be active, responsible stewards of public health data.

Adapted from: Lee, LM, Gostin, LO. Ethical collection, storage, and use of public health data: a proposal for national privacy protection. JAMA 2009;302:82–84

VII. Standards for Data Collection, Storage, Sharing, and Use to Ensure Security and Confidentiality

The following standards are based on the 10 guiding principles listed in the previous section. They represent recommended standards to ensure the security, confidentiality, and appropriate use, including sharing, of data collected by NCHHSTP-funded programs.

The standards are grouped into five topical areas: program policies and responsibilities; data collection and use; data sharing and release; physical security; and electronic data security. Each standard is followed by a brief background or explanatory statement and a set of questions to guide programs in policy development and implementation.

1.0 PROGRAM POLICIES AND RESPONSIBILITIES

STANDARD 1.1 Develop written policies and procedures on data security and confidentiality; review policies and procedures at least annually; revise them as needed; and ensure their review by and accessibility to all staff members having authorized access to confidential individual-level data.

Programs should develop and maintain written policies and procedures on data security and confidentiality. Written policies and procedures should include:

- Review of applicable laws and regulations
- Description of applicable data (include details on types of records, systems, and reports)
- Roles and responsibilities of persons with authorized access to the data
- Applicable confidentiality agreements
- Controls for data management, security, and access (physical and electronic)
- Address when use of privacy advice or reminder is appropriate (i.e., when to include privacy advice at the point of information use on forms, information collection devices, systems, file cabinets, etc.)
- Specified policies applicable to trainees, students, volunteers, visitors, and cleaning and security staff.
- Provisions to limit disclosure and prevent indirect release of PII
- Guidance on data sharing

Policies should be introduced to new staff members, students, and volunteers during orientation and reviewed with all staff members during annual training sessions. Staff members should also be notified of any changes or updates to data security policies.

See Appendix E for a suggested outline of a policy for data security, confidentiality, sharing and use.

STANDARD 1.2 Designate a person or persons to act as the overall responsible party (ORP) for the security of public health data your program collects or maintains, and ensure that the ORP is named in any policy documents related to data security.

The purpose of naming an ORP is to increase program accountability for data security. The ORP should have the authority to modify programs and policies to meet the standards in this document. The ORP can be selected from the program, section, or agency level. The agency's organizational structure might demand designating more than one person as ORP (i.e., an ORP panel). The ORP(s) may also choose to have data releases or proposed data sharing activities reviewed by a group of designated individuals to facilitate the review process and ensure the risks and benefits of the proposed activities are considered and make recommendations.

STANDARD 1.3 Ensure that data security policies define the roles and access levels of all persons with authorized access to confidential public health data and the procedures for accessing data securely.

Access to surveillance data needs to be planned. The number of people with access to identifiable information should be kept to a minimum, and de-identified data should be used for routine analyses whenever possible. Operational security procedures should be devised to minimize the number of people with access to confidential data. Written procedures should specify how to obtain authorization for access to both PII and de-identified data.

STANDARD 1.4 Ensure that data security policies require ongoing reviews of evolving technologies and include a computer back-up or disaster recovery plan.

Because the technology used to secure data is constantly evolving, information technology and security professionals should be included in the development and review of data security policies and procedures. Policies should include plans for a secondary, secure, off-site computer operation that can go into effect in the event of a catastrophic failure at the primary location. The National Institute of Standards and Technology Special Publication 800-34, Contingency Planning Guide for Federal Information Systems contains guidance on contingency planning for IT resources and is available at: http://csrc.nist.gov/publications/PubsSPs.html. [25]

> GUIDING QUESTIONS:
>
> » Have persons with technical expertise in information and system security been consulted to ensure that data security policies and procedures are adequate?
>
> » Do policies and procedures include a disaster recovery plan?

STANDARD 1.5 Ensure that any breach of data security protocol, regardless of whether personal information was released, is reported to the ORP and investigated immediately. Any breach that results in the release of PII to unauthorized persons should be reported to the ORP, to CDC, and, if warranted to law enforcement agencies.

Guidelines for a risk-based approach for protecting confidentiality of PII, including responding to breaches (incident response), are described in the National Institute of Standards and Technology Special Publication 800-122, Guide to Protecting the Confidentiality of Personally Identifiable Information available at http://csrc.nist.gov/publications/. [12] The data security policy should include procedures for reporting suspected breaches, including who to notify about a suspected breach. Staff members should be familiar with the program's definition of a security breach. Staff members should review procedures during annual security training. A log of security breaches and lessons learned during investigations of breaches might be useful in revising security policies.

Breaches that do not result in the release of PII can be handled within programs. Breaches that result in unauthorized disclosure of PII require immediate consultation with legal counsel and notification of high-level authorities in the agency to ensure appropriate action. There are federal requirements for reporting breaches of PII involving federal data or federal supported systems. For instance, based on OMB Memorandum 06-19 (http://www.whitehouse.gov/sites/default/files/omb/memoranda/fy2006/m06-19.pdf),[26] if PII from a federally supported system were to be released to, or stolen by, unauthorized persons, that breach must be reported to federal security officials within one hour of its discovery. For NCHHSTP, the designated person is the Information System Security Officer (ISSO) for the Center. Both the ISSO and the CDC program contact need to be notified immediately.

STANDARD 1.6 Ensure that staff members with access to identifiable public health data attend data security and confidentiality training annually.

All staff members (including IT personnel, contractors, and mail room and custodial staff) require generic security awareness training to ensure and support a culture of confidentiality, but staff who have access to PII require additional training specific to their responsibilities and level of authorized access to PII. Training should cover:

- Personal responsibilities
- Procedures for ensuring physical security of PII
- Procedures for electronically storing and transferring data
- Policies and procedures for data sharing
- Procedures for reporting and responding to security breaches
- Review of relevant laws and regulations

All staff should have documentation of completion of their training. Programs are responsible for maintaining this documentation in their personnel files.

STANDARD 1.7 Require all newly hired staff members to sign a confidentiality agreement before being given access to identifiable information; require all staff members to re-sign their confidentiality agreements annually.

All staff (including IT, mail room, and custodial staff) should sign a nondisclosure or confidentiality agreement stating that the employee agrees not to release PII to any unauthorized persons. The agreement should be maintained in the employee's personnel file. A confidentiality agreement should be required before assigning passwords or keys that allow access to PII. Policies and procedures should address staff out-processing and relinquishment of authorized access.

GUIDING QUESTION:

» Are all staff members required to sign a confidentiality agreement before they are granted access to PII?

STANDARD 1.8 Ensure that all persons who have authorized access to confidential public health data take responsibility for 1) implementing the program's data security policies and procedures, 2) protecting the security of any device in their possession on which PII are stored, and 3) reporting suspected security breaches.

The data security responsibilities of staff members should be incorporated into their confidentiality agreements and reviewed during annual training. Supervisors should consider including security-related questions in annual performance reviews as a way of gauging staff members' understanding of their data security responsibilities.

Responsibilities of persons with authorized access to PII include but are not limited to:

- Protecting keys, passwords, and codes that would facilitate unauthorized access to PII

- Taking appropriate action to avoid infecting computer systems with viruses and other malware

- Protecting computers and devices from extreme heat and cold

- Protecting mobile devices and storage media from loss or theft

- Appropriate use of personal computers and storage devices

- Appropriate removal of data from secure facilities

GUIDING QUESTIONS:

» Are the data security responsibilities of staff members outlined in their confidentiality agreements?

» Are these responsibilities reviewed annually?

» Are staff members aware of relevant data security policies? Have they completed security training?

» Do staff members know how, and to whom, to report suspected security breaches or instances of unauthorized access? Are they familiar with the criteria for reporting and investigation?

STANDARD 1.9 Certify annually that all data security standards have been met.

Programs should self-certify annually and work collaboratively with CDC to address any problem areas. At a minimum, programs should provide a statement that:

- Identifies the ORP

- Attests to the program's adherence to the data security standards

- Cites policies and procedures that document adherence to these standards

- Documents any reasons for non-adherence, with plans for remediation

GUIDING QUESTIONS:

» Has an ORP been named?

» Has a statement attesting to adherence to the standards been provided?

» Is a list of confidentiality and security policies and procedures available upon request?

2.0 DATA COLLECTION AND USE

STANDARD 2.1 Clearly specify the purpose for which the data will be collected.

Written policies and procedures should describe the intended public health purposes for collecting data and the scope and limits of the data collection activities when data are shared or used. A "legitimate" public health purpose includes efforts to prevent disease or premature death or promote health among members of a community through activities such as:

- Assessing the health needs and health status of a community through public health surveillance and epidemiologic research

- Developing public health policy

- Responding to public health needs and emergencies

- Evaluating public health programs

GUIDING QUESTIONS:

» What is the rationale for the proposed data collection?

» What is the intended use for the data?

» What are the limits on how the data may be used?

» Is the proposed data collection likely to lead to a reduction in morbidity and mortality rates through targeting of public health interventions without creating undue burdens?

» Is the proposed data collection significantly different from other approved public health data collection efforts?

STANDARD 2.2 Collect and use the minimum information needed to conduct specified public health activities and achieve the stated public health purpose.

Before implementing data-collection or data-sharing activities, public health practitioners should specify minimum data elements and consider whether collection and use of personally identifiable data will be necessary to achieve their public health goal.

The minimum information requirement will vary based on the activity. For example, certain personal identifiers are required for activities requiring follow-up with individuals; for partner services, that might include name and locating information such as an address, in addition to other information deemed critical for the investigation. When considering a new data-collection or data-sharing effort, consider the following guidelines:

- Specify minimum data elements, and include only the information needed to achieve the public health goal(s).

- Minimize or avoid collecting information just because it might be of later use or because it is easily accessible.

- Refer to similar high-quality data-collection efforts or data-sharing activities with proven success.

- Avoid unnecessary retention or creation of multiple data collections or data management systems (the more collections/systems, the greater the complexity of security management).

GUIDING QUESTIONS:

» What is the minimum amount of demographic, geographic, and health-related data needed to accomplish the public health goal of the proposed data collection?

» Are all proposed data elements justifiable in terms of their contribution toward achieving the public health goal?

» Are key data elements similar enough to those collected through previous data collection efforts to allow needed comparisons?

STANDARD 2.3 Collect personally identifiable data only when necessary; use nonidentifiable data whenever possible.

Identifiable data require a higher standard of protection than nonidentifiable data. Collection and use of identifiable data are justifiable if the data are to be used for a public health purpose that cannot be achieved through the use of nonidentifiable data. Published standards and recommended practices for maintaining confidentiality of PII and de-identification of data can be used to guide policy development. [12, 18, 27-32]

STANDARD 2.4 Ensure that data that are collected and/or used for public health research are done in accordance with stipulations in Common Rule, Title 45, Part 46 of the Code of Federal Regulations, which includes obtaining both institutional review board (IRB) approval for any proposed federally funded research and informed consent of individuals directly contacted for further participation.

The use of identifiable data for research is contingent on a demonstrated need for the data, IRB approval, and the signing of a confidentiality agreement regarding rules of access and final disposition of the information. The use of nonidentifiable data for research is generally permissible but might still require IRB approval, depending on the amount and type of data requested. Programs should consult applicable guidance on research versus practice and human subjects regulations.[24,33]

3.0 DATA SHARING AND RELEASE

STANDARD 3.1 Limit sharing of confidential or identifiable information to those with a justifiable public health need; ensure that any data-sharing restrictions do not compromise or impede public health program or disease surveillance activities and that the ORP or other appropriate official has approved this access.

This standard applies to the sharing of data with other public health entities that might need routine access to the data for a related public health function. For example, a TB surveillance unit and HIV unit that routinely match case registries to update case information might require some reciprocal access to each other's information. Or, a partner services program might need access to limited information on newly reported HIV cases to initiate partner services. Such access should be authorized by the ORP(s) of the program(s) maintaining the data and limited to the minimum number of persons, and amount of information necessary.

When proposing changes to policies affecting access to public health data, if the changes are significantly different from standard practices or controversial, it is good practice to first seek input from members of affected communities, medical providers, and/or other key stakeholders to ensure that the proposed changes do not adversely affect public trust in, or the integrity of, the public health system.

For any routine, authorized sharing of information, programs should verify:

- Appropriateness of sharing
- Integrity of the information shared
- Identity of the recipient
- Security of the method through which the information will be shared

GUIDING QUESTIONS:

» Is access to PII necessary to achieve a specified public health function?

» Have steps been taken to limit access to the fewest number of persons necessary?

» Is information sharing reduced to the minimum information necessary?

» Do procedures by which data will be accessed include adequate data security and confidentiality protections?

STANDARD 3.2 Assess the risks and benefits of sharing identifiable data for other than their originally stated purpose or for purposes not covered by existing policies.

Public health interventions and research often rely on the use of shared data. However, strict norms of privacy and confidentiality must govern any sharing of data, and de-identified data should be used whenever possible. Data should be shared only for legitimate public health purposes and all data sharing must comply with applicable laws and regulations. See Glossary in Appendix A for a definition of legitimate public health purposes.

Determining whether proposed data sharing is "legitimate" often involves ethical questions. An autonomous body composed of persons familiar with ethics in public health surveillance may provide insight and feedback on proposed activities.[34] Several models of ethical decision-making might provide useful, practical guidance for decisions on data use.[35-39]

- Begin by identifying the public health ethics issues in the specific situation, including those related to risks and benefits, public health goals, stakeholders, and precedent cases.

- Generate and compare different options or courses of action and the ethical rationale for each. Choose the best option and justify the chosen course of action.

- Evaluate the selected action to determine if the desired outcome was achieved.

GUIDING QUESTIONS:

» Have all alternatives to sharing such data been explored?

» Is the sharing of identifiable data necessary?

» Is the proposed use within the scope of your data-release policy and for a legitimate public health purpose?

» Have the security and confidentiality standards of the requesting party been assessed? Are the standards adequate?

» Does the entity receiving identifiable data have in place confidentiality and security standards that meet the standards outlined in this document?

STANDARD 3.3 Ensure that any public health program with which personally identifiable public health data are shared has data security standards equivalent to those in this document.

Confidentiality can be compromised if data are shared with programs that lack adequate security and confidentiality protections.

- Share data only after the ORP(s) has weighed the benefits and risks of allowing access.

- Share data only with programs that have written policies and procedures establishing data security and confidentiality protections equivalent to those in this document.

GUIDING QUESTIONS:

» Does the program accessing the data have written security and confidentiality policies and procedures?

» Have the policies and procedures been reviewed and found to be consistent with the standards in this document?

STANDARD 3.4 Ensure that public health information is released only for purposes related to public health, except where required by law.

Programs should establish data release policies and procedures that delineate any exceptional circumstances that may warrant the release of identifiable data and how the confidentiality of such data will be protected. Programs can develop routine disclosure procedures that outline a process for reviewing routine disclosures.[40] Review procedures could include designating a group of persons, including the ORP(s) to review nonroutine data releases. Before allowing nonroutine disclosures, policies could include a brief period of contemplation, or timeout, before releasing data to minimize risk of improper disclosure.[40]

Programs should not release PII to anyone outside of public health except in circumstances involving significant risk of harm to the public or if required by law. Even when required, only the minimum information should be released. The ORP and legal counsel of the program(s) controlling the data should review any request for PII to determine the specific data, if any, that must be released. In some instances, the information requested may be available from other sources. When information is ordered for release as part of a judicial proceeding, any release or discussion of information should occur in closed judicial proceedings, if possible.

GUIDING QUESTIONS:

» Is the release of identifiable data to officials in law enforcement, immigration control, or public welfare management justified by an imminent threat to individuals or populations or other compelling circumstances?

» Have all possible alternatives to the use of identifiable data been examined before the release of such data?

» Has a legal analysis been conducted by the health department's legal counsel?

» What non-public health use of the data is required or allowed by law?

STANDARD 3.5 Establish procedures, including assessment of risks and benefits, for determining whether to grant requests for aggregate data not covered by existing data-release policies.

Procedures could include a process designating a group of persons to review requests that are outside the stated policy. Any data release must be for a legitimate public health purpose and in accordance with applicable laws and regulations.

GUIDING QUESTION:

» Are there precedents for the requested release of data? If so, how were those precedent cases handled?

STANDARD 3.6 Disseminate nonidentifiable summary data to stakeholders as soon as possible after data are collected.

Written policies should address procedures for the dissemination of nonidentifiable summary data to stakeholders and the public. Summary data should be disseminated in a manner that facilitates understanding by affected populations and illuminates the compounding impact of syndemics.

Since some aggregate data could be used to identify individuals, policies should usually restrict release of certain data elements to avoid a confidentiality breach. Wider public access and searchability of databases (e.g., death records and obituaries) increases the capability to re-identify other de-identified data. Consideration should be given to consulting with de-identification experts prior to release when in doubt. In some instances, the obligation to use the data to help members of demographic groups examine trends and burden of disease for public health planning might outweigh the risk of possible stigma that could be associated with some aggregate data. For example, the release of data showing high rates of alcohol and drug use in a small community, although potentially stigmatizing, must be weighed against the potential additional resource planning and allocation for drug and alcohol treatment services that could result from such a release.

GUIDING QUESTIONS:

» Have data dissemination plans been described? What efforts have been made to ensure that nonidentifiable data are disseminated regularly and in a timely manner?

» Are procedures in place to assess the usefulness of data dissemination efforts?

» What precautions have been taken to ensure that the disseminated data are not presented in ways that may indirectly identify individuals?

STANDARD 3.7 Assess data quality before disseminating data.

Evaluations of data quality should occur during collection, management, analysis, and use to ensure sufficiently accurate and valid data. The quality of public health data is critical to the validity of public health policies and actions based on these data.

Guidance on ensuring data quality is provided in the HHS Guidelines for Ensuring the Quality of Information Disseminated to the Public, Part D, CDC and the Agency for Toxic Substances and Disease Registry (ATSDR). Quality assurance mechanisms described in the document include internal reviews, external reviews, merit reviews, and peer reviews. Programs may also consult with independent researchers and experts in areas such as data collection and data analysis; maintain ongoing contact with data users and participate in conferences and workshops to assess the needs of potential data users; and use a wide variety of dissemination mechanisms to make statistical and analytic information broadly accessible.[41]

STANDARD 3.8 Ensure that data-release policies define purposes for which the data can be used and provisions to prevent public access to raw data or data tables that could contain indirectly identifying information.

The main challenge in developing responsible data-release policies is to balance the need to make data available to a broad audience and in a timely manner with the need to protect individual privacy. Data-release policies should address:

- Purpose and types of data (e.g., de-identified, patient-level, and aggregate) that can be released
- Intended audience
- Rules for suppression
- Rules for dissemination of aggregate data products
- Physical and electronic (including IT) controls to ensure data security
- Mechanisms and procedures for requesting data and considering data requests
- Suggested formats for data-use agreements

Useful standards for data-release and data-sharing reflect principles and policies outlined in the CDC/ATSDR Policy on Releasing and Sharing Data,[13] the CDC-CSTE Intergovernmental Data Release Guidelines Working Group Report: CDC/ATSDR Data Release Guidelines and Procedures for Re-release of State-Provided Data.[4] The CDC/ATSDR policy provides guidance aimed at balancing the desire to disseminate data as broadly as possible with the need to maintain high standards and protect confidential information, while also ensuring compliance with applicable federal regulations and guidelines. The Office of Management and Budget's (OMB) Federal Committee on Statistical Methodology, Statistical Policy Working Paper 22: Report on Statistical Disclosure Limitation Methodology also provides useful guidance for developing data release policies.[31]

GUIDING QUESTIONS:

» Do the data-release policies address the following?

- Roles and responsibilities of program personnel, including any confidentiality agreements they must sign and any training they must receive

- Access procedures and authorization rules

- Descriptions of the data and to whom, and in what format, they can be released

- Procedures for data release

- Specific requirements for sharing identifiable data

- Mechanisms for data release, including rules for minimizing disclosure such as cell-size restrictions

- Disposition of data after they have been used for a stated purpose

» Do data release plans include mechanisms for evaluating the usefulness of released data and whether the release of data is causing undue burden on individuals or communities?

4.0 PHYSICAL SECURITY

STANDARD 4.1 To the extent possible, ensure that persons working with hard copies of documents containing confidential, identifiable information do so in a secure, locked area.

Physical access controls should be in place to protect hard-copy data and computer equipment. Operational security procedures should be devised to minimize the number of storage locations in which PII is held.

Minimum Secure Area

- Work space with limited access for only necessary staff
- Locked file cabinets that are large and heavy enough to render them immobile
- A designated location within the work space where confidential conversations may be held

Enhanced Security Configurations

- A dedicated, secure area accessible only via locked door with limited key or keycard distribution to minimal staff
- Double-locked file cabinets that are large and heavy enough to render them immobile
- A workstation/table equipped with a telephone and computer to handle data within the secure space

A dedicated, secure room would be the preferred location for confidential, secured data stored in locked, immobile cabinets. Additionally, this space could provide a table or work station for staff to conduct confidential telephone conversations. In the absence of a dedicated, secure room, a reasonable alternative could be an area which is accessible only from within the surveillance area to house immobile, locked file cabinets. If necessary, one secure file cabinet could be shared by several small programs within a jurisdiction if they have the same data security standards.

If data must be stored or used in less than ideally secure work areas, the security of these areas should be improved as much as possible. For example, in many workplaces confidentiality is improved by requiring paper documents with confidential information to be kept locked in desk drawers when not in use or when a worker is away from his or her desk. Security might also be improved by reconfiguring cubicles, office partitions, and requiring confidential phone conversations to take place in a private room. This is not an exhaustive list of improvements, but it shows that creative thinking may be needed to turn an open work area into a more secure workplace.

In the course of public health work, and in the evolving modern work environment, confidential data may be handled not only outside the secure work area, but off-site, in the field, or in telework/remote sites (see Appendix G for guidelines on working in nontraditional settings).

It is critical that project areas develop and implement protocols for telework, remote work, and field work, in addition to core confidentiality and security policies. Even if these work activities have not yet been implemented in a project area, provisions should be made for their future implementation by including them in the current protocols.

STANDARD 4.2 Ensure that documents containing confidential information are shredded with crosscutting shredders before disposal.

Crosscutting features are needed to ensure confidential information cannot be recovered. See National Institute of Standards and Technology Special Publication 800-88, Guidelines for Media Sanitation, available at http://csrc.nist.gov/publications/, for discussion of shredding and destruction of paper and other media.[42] Contracting with a document-shredding service may be an option for some programs. If a service is used, be sure that documents are shredded on site and in the presence of a staff member. In all cases, a contract shredding or disposal company must be bonded, and due diligence should be taken in the selection of the company.

STANDARD 4.3 Ensure that data-security policies and procedures address handling of paper copies, incoming and outgoing mail, long-term paper storage, and data retention. The amount of confidential information in all such correspondence should be kept to a minimum and destroyed when no longer needed.

Policies should address retention of paper copies. If electronic copies exist, paper copies can be destroyed when no longer needed, in accordance with established health department policies. Provisions should be made to destroy copies using methods described in Standard 4.2.

STANDARD 4.4 Limit access to secure areas that contain confidential public health data to authorized persons, and establish procedures to control access to secure areas by non-authorized persons.

Data security policies and procedures should specify who has access to secure areas. Policies and procedures must also address the need for access by unauthorized persons (e.g., cleaning, maintenance, and security staff). Programs might consider providing cleaning crews with access to secure areas only when authorized staff members are present or when confidential materials are stored and protected.

GUIDING QUESTIONS:

» Do policies adequately describe who has access to secure areas?

» Do data security policies and procedures address access to secure areas and file storage areas by cleaning crews and maintenance staff?

» Are procedures in place to control access to secure areas by other unauthorized personnel?

STANDARD 4.5 Ensure that program personnel working with documents containing PII in the field 1) return the documents to a secure area by close of business, 2) obtain prior approval from the program manager for not doing so, or 3) follow approved procedures for handling such documents.

Simple physical theft is a major cause of health information breaches. Transportation and use of PII outside of secure areas should, therefore, be minimized and carefully controlled. Programs employing field workers should establish specific procedures for:

- Working with PII outside of secure areas

- Obtaining or documenting a manager's approval to do so

- Physically securing documents containing PII that remain in staff custody after usual work hours

GUIDING QUESTIONS:

» Do policies include procedures for securing documents containing PII when they cannot be returned to a secure work site by the close of business?

» Do policies outline specific reasons, permissions and physical security procedures for using, transporting and protecting documents containing PII in a vehicle or personal residence?

STANDARD 4.6 Ensure that documents with line lists or supporting notes contain the minimum amount of potentially identifiable information [PII] necessary and, if possible, that any potentially identifiable data are coded to prevent inadvertent release of PII.

To the extent possible, PII should not be removed from a secure location or accessed from an unsecure area. However, some public health activities (e.g., field investigations and service provision) require taking such information into unsecure areas. In these situations, the use of PII should be limited and appropriate security measures implemented.

GUIDING QUESTIONS:

» Is access to public health notes and investigation information containing identifiable data limited to personnel requiring the information for an approved purpose?

» Are confidential data elements coded?

5.0 ELECTRONIC DATA SECURITY

Implementation of electronic data security standards will be conducted in a rapidly evolving technological environment. While technology is changing, the following elements will remain important to consider when developing policies.

Access: Access to surveillance data needs to be planned in advance. Access groups can be set up in virtually all IT environments, which will allow the program to designate users with different levels and types of rights. Programs should specify who has access to various data, under what circumstances, and how the identity of users are authenticated. For example, they might stipulate that identifiable data should be accessed only from a properly secure network server rather than from local workstations. Isolated segments or domains can be implemented, which limits access to those in selected groups. They also might limit the times during which data can be accessed, restrict the copying or downloading of data, and set up other controls as needed. Due to the technical nature of these control measures, IT personnel should be involved in the initial assessment and both the formulation and implementation of electronic data security policies. *Appendix G also addresses electronic data security issues.*

Encryption and Backups: Although encryption may not be needed for data on a production registry or surveillance data system located within a secure area and separate from any networks, encryption is still recommended. Any data in such a registry or system do need to be encrypted before being transmitted or downloaded to approved locations and while being used in the field on laptops or similar devices. Although surveillance databases and other files with identifying information need to be backed up, back-up databases and files should be encrypted in accordance with federal encryption standards and stored in a secure location. Bonded storage companies can be used to store back-up files of identifiable data as long as the data are encrypted according to standard operating procedures. Encryption is one means of increasing data security. Backup data should also be encrypted before being copied to a secure location. All encryption methods need to meet standards detailed in Federal Information Processing Standards (FIPS) Publication 197, Advanced Encryption Standard (AES). (See http://csrc.nist.gov/publications/fips/fips197/fips-197.pdf.) [43]

Evolving Technologies: Many public health workers handle PII in the field while pursuing public health activities, and as technology continues to evolve, use of PDAs, electronic tablets, and notebook computers may involve data stored on portable devices. Programs must therefore plan for migration from paper-oriented to electronic systems that meet established and evolving electronic and procedural security standards. Forward-looking confidentiality and security protocols should include provisions for phones, PDAs, tablets, and workbooks that take client-identified data to the field and allow for real-time updates, reporting, and data entry from field sites as well as by medical staff in examination rooms. These protocols should also provide accountability measures to ensure that staff members employ this secured, confidential data in appropriate locations while in the field. Programs may review National Institute of Standards and Technology Special Publication 800-124, Guidelines on Cell Phone and PDA Security, available at http://csrc.nist.gov/publications/) when developing policies. [44]

Surveillance programs will be increasingly using electronic medical records and electronic laboratory records to complete case reports. Many health departments already have or are considering public health information exchanges which have the potential to enhance surveillance data collections. When implementing these activities programs should ensure secure methods are used and policies and procedures ensure security and confidentiality of data. Additional resources on electronic data exchange can be found at http://www.cdc.gov/ehrmeaningfuluse/ and the public health information network (http://www.cdc.gov/phin/).

Secure Transmission: Data to be transmitted across defined, secure boundaries should be transmitted through the use of secure methods, such as secure data networks (SDNs), virtual private networks (VPNs), and secure file transport protocol (SFTP). Although these methods can be used to encrypt data in transit, they do not encrypt data before they are sent or after they are received. Therefore, if either the sender or the recipient of the data is not part of a defined security zone appropriate for sensitive data, data should be encrypted by another method prior to being transmitted. Since transmission of data via cell phones or PDAs is similarly insecure, identifiable information should also not be sent with these devices.

STANDARD 5.1 Ensure that analysis data sets that can be accessed from outside the secure area are stored with protective software (i.e., software that controls data storage, removal, and use), and verify removal of all personal identifiers.

Analysis data sets should be stored on a separate server or segmented local area network (LAN). At a minimum, analysis data sets should be located on a virtual server and all personal identifiers should be removed. The inclusion of sensitive or potentially linkable data elements such as a lab ID, accession number, or case report number should be limited to those required for analysis and should not be included in analysis data sets. Given the increasing ability to re-identify records by matching between multiple publically accessible databases, consultation with a de-identification expert may be useful before making de-identified databases publically available.

Encryption of analysis data sets, when not in use, is not necessary if personally identifiable data elements have been removed. However, encryption is recommended as additional protection from accidental or purposeful misuse.

GUIDING QUESTIONS:

» Are roles assigned to selected individuals to create analysis data sets to minimize the number created?

» What measures have been taken to ensure that analysis data sets are created, stored, and accessed securely?

» Do data security policies describe the data elements that may be included in analysis data sets?

STANDARD 5.2 Ensure that any electronic transfer of data is approved by the ORP and subject to access controls, and that identifiable data are encrypted before being transferred.

This standard applies particularly to situations in which data are obtained electronically from sources outside the health department (e.g., electronic laboratory data, electronic health records, Web-based systems, hospitals, and other large providers). Extracts from these systems should meet the minimum security standards outlined in this document. Electronic records should be protected through security devices such as sign-on passwords, encryption, and audit trails. External sources should be encouraged to review their procedures. Approved data transfer methods should be used when designing electronic reporting mechanisms for laboratories, providers, etc.

As possible, data with PII should be encrypted while in transit and when at rest. Ideally, data-transfers should be done over a secure data network (SDN), virtual private network (VPN) connection with certificates on both the sending and the receiving ends, or similar secure connection. At a minimum, data transfer should be performed via a secure application such as a file transfer protocol (FTP) for which certification is required on at least one end.

Electronic files being stored for future use (e.g., ancillary data and working laboratory data sets) should be encrypted until needed. If these files are needed outside the secure area, use of real-time encryption or an equivalent method of protection is recommended.

GUIDING QUESTIONS:

» Are routine electronic transfers of data containing identifiable data done through secure methods, and are data encrypted before transfer?

» Are encryption methods that meet Advanced Encryption Standards (AES) always used to move identifiable public health data? (See http://csrc.nist.gov/publications/fips/fips197/fips-197.pdf.)

» Are ancillary or working data sets containing PII encrypted when not in use?

STANDARD 5.3 Before transferring electronic data containing PII, ensure that the data have been encrypted with use of an encryption package that meets Advanced Encryption Standard (AES) criteria and that the data transfer has been approved by the appropriate program official or ORP. No electronic data containing identifying information should be transferred without being encrypted.

PII must be safeguarded to maintain confidentiality. The preferred method of securing data is with whole-device encryption that fulfills FIPS 140-2 standards available at http://csrc.nist.gov/publications/fips/fips140-2/fips1402.pdf. Device encryption ensures that "remnants" of any files that were opened or deleted from the device are fully secure. File encryption is adequate only when used in connection with proper physical protections. The least appropriate security measure is to rely totally on physical protection and should be used only in highly secure and restricted environments. The decision to use physical protections over an encryption solution is a risk-based decision, as these protections cannot completely remove the risk of theft or loss of sensitive data.

Confidential, individual-level public health data should be transferred via more secure electronic transfer methods, personal communication, or hard-copy mail delivery when at all possible. At a minimum, programs that choose to fax paper documents containing PII should take steps to make it as secure as possible. Partners who submit identifiable data to health departments also need to be informed of acceptable methods of transfer. Guidelines for the use of facsimile machines are included in Appendix F.

E-mailing of unencrypted personally identifiable information is not allowed. Unintended release of confidential unencrypted e-mail may result. E-mail inadvertently might be sent to an unintended recipient, and even an encrypted e-mail might result in unintended access. Health departments must also adhere to relevant "sunshine" laws regarding access to government e-mails. If public access to e-mail is required, the process of publicly contesting the release of information is not likely to play out well to the general public.

GUIDING QUESTIONS:

» Has identifying information been removed from unencrypted data before they are transferred electronically?

» Are encryption methods that meet AES standards always used in the transfer of identifiable data?

» Are procedures in place for limiting faxing of confidential data? If faxes are used, what additional procedures are in place to secure the information and ensure that it is sent to the intended recipient only?

» Do data policies address e-mailing of public health data?

» Is identifying information always removed from data or encrypted prior to the data being sent by e-mail?

STANDARD 5.4 Use encryption software that meets federal AES standards to encrypt data with PII on all laptops and other portable devices that receive or store public health data with personal identifiers.

PII on a laptop must be encrypted and stored on an external storage device or removable hard drive. The external storage device or hard drive containing the data must be separated from the laptop and held securely when not in use. The decryption key must not be on the laptop. Portable devices without removable or external storage components must have encryption software that meets federal AES standards. All removable or external storage devices containing identifiable public health data must:

- Include only the minimum amount of information necessary to accomplish assigned tasks as determined by the designated official or ORP

- Be encrypted or stored under lock and key when not in use

- Be sanitized immediately following a given task (except for those used as back-ups)

Before any portable device containing sensitive data is removed from a secure area, the data must be encrypted. Methods used to sanitize a storage device must ensure that any data on the device cannot be retrieved by using "undelete" or data retrieval software. Hard drives, flash drives, or any other storage media of computers that once contained PII must be sanitized or physically destroyed before the computers are labeled as excess or surplus, reassigned to other staff members, or sent off-site for repair. This requirement also applies to copiers, printers, fax machines, or other equipment that contain internal storage devices.

GUIDING QUESTIONS:

» Do policies describe when PII may be stored on external devices?

» Are stored data appropriately encrypted?

» Do policies describe how to sanitize or physically destroy storage devices when tasks are completed?

» Do policies restrict use of photographic and video devices in areas containing PII, especially in areas where there are paper documents? Do policies explicitly include cell phones and PDAs with picture and video storage capability?

STANDARD 5.5 Ensure that data policies include procedures for handling incoming and outgoing facsimile transmissions. Minimize inclusion of PII in fax transmissions, and destroy hard copies and sanitize hard drives when no longer needed.

- The faxing of identifiable information is allowed but should be avoided when possible (see Appendix F for guidelines on the use of facsimile machines). The sender of a fax cannot be certain that the fax will actually be received by the person for whom it was intended. Although encrypted fax machines are available, they would be needed at both ends of an encrypted fax transmission.

- When a fax is necessary, minimize inclusion of confidential information.

- Take precautions (such as a telephone call) to ensure that the recipient is present to receive, and confirm receipt of, the fax.

GUIDING QUESTIONS:

» Have all alternatives to faxing PII been explored?

» Have confidential data items been kept to a minimum?

» Have steps been taken to ensure that a person is standing by to receive and confirm receipt of a fax containing PII?

» Have the steps in Appendix F been followed to ensure secure use of fax machines?

VIII. References

1. Weinstock H, Douglas JM Jr, Fenton KA. Toward integration of STD, HIV, TB, and viral hepatitis surveillance. *Public Health Rep.* 2009;124(Suppl 2):5–6.

2. Gostin LO, Lazzarini Z, Neslund VS, Osterholm MT. The public health information infrastructure: a national review of the law on health information privacy. *JAMA* 1996;275:1921–1927.

3. O'Connor, J, Matthews G. Informational Privacy, Public Health, and State Laws. *AJPH.* 2011;101(10):1845-1850.

4. CDC-CSTE Intergovernmental Data Release Guidelines Working Group. CDC/ATSDR Data Release Guidelines and Procedures for Re-release of State-Provided Data. http://www.cste.org/dnn/Portals/0/drgwgreport.pdf. Accessed November 14-2011.

5. Delcher PC, Edwards KT, Stover JA, Newman LM, Groseclose SL, Rajnik DM. Data suppression strategies used during surveillance data release by sexually transmitted disease prevention programs. *J Public Health Manag Pract.* 2008;14:E1–E8.

6. Centers for Disease Control and Prevention. Program Collaboration and Service Integration: Enhancing the Prevention and Control of HIV/AIDS, Viral Hepatitis, Sexually Transmitted Diseases, and Tuberculosis in the United States. http://www.cdc.gov/nchhstp/programintegration/docs/207181-C_NCHHSTP_PCSI%20WhitePaper-508c.pdf. Accessed November 14, 2011.

7. Centers for Disease Control and Prevention. NCHHSTP external consultation on program collaboration and service integration: meeting report summary. http://www.cdc.gov/nchhstp/programintegration/docs/PCSImeetingreportwithcover11-26%20_2.pdf. Effective November 2007. Accessed November 14, 2011.

8. Centers for Disease Control and Prevention. *Guidelines for HIV/AIDS Surveillance.* Appendix C: Security and Confidentiality. Atlanta, GA: Centers for Disease Control and Prevention, US Dept of Health and Human Services; 1998.

9. Centers for Disease Control and Prevention, Council of State and Territorial Epidemiologists. *Technical Guidance for HIV/AIDS Surveillance Programs, Volume III: Security and confidentiality guidelines.* Atlanta, GA: Centers for Disease Control and Prevention, 2006.

10. Frieden TR, Das-Douglas M, Kellerman SE, Henning KJ. Applying public health principles to the HIV epidemic. *N Engl J Med.* 2005;353:2397-2402.

11. Centers for Disease Control and Prevention. Recommendations for partner services programs for HIV infection, syphilis, gonorrhea, and chlamydial infection. *MMWR Morb Mortal Wkly Rep.* 2008;57(RR-9): 1-63.

12. National Institute of Standards and Technology. *Guide to Protecting the Confidentiality of Personally Identifiable Information.* Gaithersburg, MD: National Institute of Standards and Technology, US Dept of Commerce; 2009.

13. Centers for Disease Control and Prevention, Agency for Toxic Substances and Disease Registry. CDC/ATSDR *Policy on Releasing and Sharing Data*. Atlanta, GA: Centers for Disease Control and Prevention, US Dept of Health and Human Services; 2005.

14. Gostin LO, Hodge JG, Valdiserri RO. Informational privacy and the public's health: the Model State Public Health Privacy Act. *Am J Public Health*. 2001;91:1388-1392.

15. Gostin LO, Hodge JG. The Model State Public Health Privacy Act. 1999. http://www.publichealthlaw.net/ModelLaws/MSPHPA.php. Updated January 27, 2010. Accessed November 14, 2011.

16. Public Health Statute Modernization Collaborative. Model State Public Health Act: A Tool for Assessing Public Health Laws. http://www.turningpointprogram.org/Pages/pdfs/statute_mod/MSPHAfinal.pdf. Effective September 2003. Accessed November 14, 2011.

17. Hodge JG, Gostin LO, Gebbie K, Erickson DL. Transforming public health law: the Turning Point Model State Public Health Act. *J Law Med Ethics*. 2006;34:77-84.

18. US Department of Health and Human Services. Health Insurance Portability and Accountability Act of 1996 (HIPAA) Privacy Rules. http://www.hhs.gov/ocr/hipaa/. Accessed November 14, 2011.

19. Fairchild AL, Gable L, Gostin LO, Bayer R, Sweeney P, Janssen RS. Public goods, private data: HIV and the history, ethics, and uses of identifiable public health information. *Public Health Rep*. 2007;122(Suppl 1):7-15.

20. Heilig CM, Sweeney P. Ethics in Public Health Surveillance. In: Lee LM, Teutsch SM, Thacker SB, St Louis ME, eds. *Principles and Practice of Public Health Surveillance*. Oxford University Press; 2010:198-216.

21. Lee, LM, Gostin, LO. Ethical collection, storage, and use of public health data: a proposal for national privacy protection. *JAMA*. 2009;302:82-84.

22. Thomas JC, Sage M, Dillenberg J, Guillory VJ. A code of ethics for public health. *Am J of Public Health*. 2002;92(7):1057–1059.

23. Public Health Leadership Society. Principles of the ethical practice of public health. Version 2.2. http://www.apha.org/NR/rdonlyres/1CED3CEA-287E-4185-9CBD-BD405FC60856/0/ethicsbrochure.pdf. Effective 2002. Accessed November 14, 2011.

24. US Department of Health and Human Services. Federal policy for the protection of human subjects (CFR Title 45, Part 46). http://www.hhs.gov/ohrp/humansubjects/guidance/45cfr46.html. Revised January 15, 2009. Effective July 14, 2009. Accessed November 14, 2011.

25. Swanson M, Bowen P, Phillips AW, Gallup D, Lynes; National Institute of Standards and Technology. National Institute of Standards and Technology Special Publication 800-34 Rev. 1, *Contingency Planning Guide for Federal Information Systems*. Gaithersburg, MD: National Institute of Standards and Technology, US Dept of Commerce; 2009.

26. Office of Management and Budget. OMB Memorandum 06-19. http://www.whitehouse.gov/sites/default/files/omb/memoranda/fy2006/m06-19.pdf. Effective July 12, 2006. Accessed November 14, 2011.

27. Committee on the Role of Institutional Review Boards in Health Services Research Data Privacy Protection. *Protecting Data Privacy in Health Services Research*. Washington, DC: Division of Health Care Services, Institute of Medicine; 2000.

28. Doyle P, Lane J, Theeuwes J, Zayatz L, eds. *Confidentiality, disclosure and data access: theory and practical applications for statistical agencies.* New York: North Holland; 2001.

29. *Record Linkage and Privacy: Issues in Creating New Federal Research and Statistical Information.* No. GAO-01-126SP. Washington, DC: Government Accountability Office; 2001.

30. Confidentiality and Data Access Committee. *Identifiability in Microdata Files.* Washington, DC: Office of Management and Budget; 2002.

31. Federal Committee on Statistical Methodology. Report on Statistical Disclosure Limitation Methodology (Statistical Working Paper 22). Washington, DC: Office of Management and Budget; 2005.

32. Yasnoff W. Privacy, confidentiality, and security of public health information. In: O'Carroll PW, Yasnoff WA, Ward ME, Ripp LH, Martin EL, eds. *Public Health Informatics and Information Systems.* New York, NY: Springer Publication; 2003.

33. Hodge JG, Gostin LO; Council of State and Territorial Epidemiologists Advisory Committee. Public Health Practice vs. Research. http://www.cste.org/pdffiles/newpdffiles/CSTEPHResRptHodgeFinal.5.24.04.pdf, Effective May 24, 2004. Accessed November 14, 2011.

34. Baily MA, Bottrell M, Lynn J, Jennings B. The ethics of using QI methods to improve health care quality and safety. *Hastings Cent Rep* 2006;36:S1–S40.

35. Childress JF, Faden RR, Gaare RD, et al. Public Health Ethics: Mapping the Terrain. *J Law Med Ethics.* 2002;30:170-178.

36. Kass NE. An Ethics Framework for Public Health. *Am J Public Health.* 2001;91:1776-1782.

37. Bernheim RG, Nieburg P, Bonnie RJ. Ethics and the practice of public health. In: Goodman RA, ed. *Law in Public Health Practice.* 2nd ed. New York, NY: Oxford University Press; 2007.

38. Roberts MJ, Reich MR. Ethical Analysis in Public Health. *Lancet.* 2002;359:1055-1059.

39. Centers for Disease Control and Prevention, Public Health Ethics Committee. *Ethics Consults in Public Health.* Atlanta, GA: Centers for Disease Control and Prevention; 2009.

40. Myers J, Frieden TR, Bherwani, KM, Henning KJ. Privacy and public health at risk: public health confidentiality in the digital age. *Am J Public Health.* 2008;98:793-801.

41. Centers for Disease Control and Prevention, Agency for Toxic Substances and Disease Registry. Guidelines for ensuring the quality of information disseminated to the public. http://www.cdc.gov/maso/qualitycontrol/Guidelines.htm, Accessed November 11, 2011.

42. Kissel R, Scholl M, Skolochenko S, Xing L; National Institute of Standards and Technology. National Institute of Standards and Technology Special Publication 800-88, *Guidelines for Media Sanitization.* Gaithersburg, MD: National Institute of Standards and Technology, US Dept of Commerce; 2006.

43. National Institute of Standards and Technology. Federal Information Processing Standards Publication 197, *Advanced Encryption Standard (AES).* Gaithersburg, MD: National Institute of Standards and Technology, US Dept of Commerce; 2001.

44. National Institute of Standards and Technology. Special Publication 800-124, *Guidelines on Cell Phone and PDA Security.* Gaithersburg, MD: National Institute of Standards and Technology, US Dept of Commerce; 2008.

Acknowledgements

External Consultants to the NCHHSTP Surveillance Work Group

Nanette Benbow Chicago Department of Public Health, STI/HIV Division

Barbara Conrad Maryland Dept of Health & Mental Hygiene

Maria Courogen Washington State Department of Health

Kim Field National Tuberculosis Controllers Association; Washington Department of Health

Douglas Frye Los Angeles County Department of Health

Elena Rizzo New York State Department of Health/Communicable Disease Control

Ann Robbins Texas Department of State Health Services

Michael Samuel California Department of Public Health, STD Control Branch

Karla Schmitt Florida Department of Health, Bureau of STD

Stanley See Texas Department of State Health Services, TB/HIV/STD Epidemiology & Surveillance

Sandra Serna-Smith National Coalition of STD Directors

Linda Lou Smith New York State Department of Health, Bureau of HIV/AIDS Epidemiology

Mark Stenger Washington State Department of Health

Lucia Torian New York City Department of Health

Amy Warner Colorado Department of Public Health and Environment

Kathy Watt Urban Coalition on HIV/AIDS Prevention Services

Janice Westenhouse California Department of Health

Elizabeth Zeringue North Carolina Department of Health and Human Services

Appendix A. Glossary

Access: Ability or means needed to read, write, modify, or communicate data/information.

Access control: Cohesive set of procedures designed to ensure that anyone with access to identifiable public health data:
- Is the person he or she claims to be (authentication),
- Has a verified public health need to have access to the data in question, and
- Has been authorized to access the data and is doing so from an authorized place using an authorized process

Advanced Encryption Standard (AES): This standard specifies the algorithm that can be used to protect electronic data and is issued by the National Institute of Standards and Technology (NIST). Publication 197 of the Federal Information Processing Standards (FIPS) (http://csrc.nist.gov/publications/fips/fips197/fips-197.pdf) contains the specifications of the AES, which can encrypt (encipher) and decrypt (decipher) information. Encryption converts data to an unintelligible form called cipher text; decrypting the cipher text converts the data back to its original form, called plaintext. The AES algorithm is capable of using cryptographic keys of 128, 192, and 256 bits to encrypt and decrypt data in blocks of 128 bits. NIST publication 140-2 details the protection of a cryptographic module within a security system necessary to maintain the confidentiality and integrity of the information protected by the module http://csrc.nist.gov/publications/fips/fips140-2/fips1402.pdf.

Aggregated data: Information—usually summary statistics—that might be compiled from personally identifiable information (PII) but is grouped so as to preclude identification of individual persons.

Analysis dataset: Set of aggregated data created by removing identifying information (e.g., names, addresses, ZIP codes, telephone numbers) so that the data cannot be linked to a specific person but can still be used for data analysis.

Authorized access: As determined by the ORP or designee, permission granted to an authorized person to see confidential or potentially identifiable public health data, based on the public health role of the individual and their need to know.

Authorized person: Person who has been granted authorized access to confidential information to carry out assigned duties and for whom a current, signed, approved, and binding nondisclosure agreement is on file.

Breach: A departure from established policies or procedures, or a compromise, unauthorized disclosure, unauthorized acquisition, unauthorized access, or loss of control of personally identifiable information (PII). A breach is an infraction or violation of a policy, standard, obligation, or law. A breach in data security would include any unauthorized use of data, even aggregated data without names. A breach may be malicious or unintentional.

Breach of confidentiality: A breach, as defined above, that results in the release of PII to unauthorized persons (i.e., employees or members of the general public).

Breach of Personally Identifiable Information: Defined by OMB Memorandum 07-16, Safeguarding Against and Responding to the Breach of Personally Identifiable Information, to include the loss of control, compromise, unauthorized disclosure, unauthorized acquisition, unauthorized access, or any similar term referring to situations where persons other than authorized users and for an other than authorized purpose have access or potential access to personally identifiable information, whether physical or electronic.

Confidential information: Any private information about an identifiable person who has not given consent to make that information public.

Confidentiality: Protection of personal information collected by public health organizations. The right to such protection is based on the principle that personal information should not be released without the consent of the person involved except as necessary to protect public health.

Confidentiality agreement (or nondisclosure agreement): A contract between at least two parties that outlines confidential material, knowledge, or information that the parties wish to share with one another for certain purposes, but wish to restrict access to by third parties. It is a contract through which the parties agree not to further disclose information covered by the agreement.

Data dissemination: Any mechanism by which data (typically in aggregate form) are made available to users. Includes mechanisms whereby data are released to users as well as mechanisms whereby data are made available without being released.

Data encryption standard (DES): Algorithm that encrypts and decrypts data in 64-bit blocks. Since the DES always operates on data blocks of equal size and uses both permutations and substitutions in its algorithm, it is both a block cipher and a product cipher.

Data sharing: Granting certain individuals or organizations access to data that contain personally identifiable information with the understanding that personally identifiable or potentially identifiable data cannot be re-released further unless a special data-sharing agreement governs the use and re-release of the data and is agreed upon by the receiving program and the data provider(s).

Data-sharing agreement: Mechanism by which a data requestor and data provider can define the terms of data access that can be granted to requestors.

Data release: Dissemination of data either in a public-use file or as a result of an ad hoc request which results in the data steward no longer controlling the use of the data. Data may be released in a variety of formats including, but not limited to, tables, microdata (person records), or online query systems.

Data steward: Person responsible for ensuring that data used or stored in an organization's computer systems are secure, classified appropriately, and used in accordance with organizational policies.

Disaster recovery: Use of off-site computer operations (where copies of data and information systems are stored) to recover data lost as the result of a catastrophe at the primary site of data storage or to activate information systems to replace those lost.

Disclosure: Occurs when identifiable information concerning an individual is made known to a third party. Disclosures may be *authorized* (as when a person has consented to the information being so divulged), *unauthorized* (as when information is intentionally revealed to a party not consented to by the person), or *inadvert* (as when a tabulation or file is unintentionally made available to the public that reveals or can be used to reveal personal information).

Encryption: Manipulation or encoding of information so that only parties intended to view the information can do so. The most commonly available encryption systems involve public key and symmetric key cryptography. In general, for both public and symmetric systems, the larger the key, the more robust the protection.

Identifiable data or identifiable information: See *Personally identifiable information.*

Information security: Protection of data against unauthorized access. Effective security measures are always a balance between technology and personnel management.

Legitimate public health purpose (see also public health data use): Population-based activity or individual effort aimed primarily at the prevention of injury, disease, or premature mortality. This term also refers to the promotion of health in the community, including: 1) assessing the health needs and status of the community through public health surveillance and epidemiologic research; 2) developing public health policy; and 3) responding to public health needs and emergencies. Public health purposes can include analysis and evaluation of conditions of public health importance and evaluation of public health programs.

Management controls: Controls that include policies for operating information technology resources and for authorizing the capture, processing, storage, and transmission of various types of information. They also may include training of staff, oversight, and appropriate and vigorous response to infractions.

Need-to-know access: Access to data granted to a specific person on a case-specific basis where exceptional circumstances exist that are not stipulated in program policies. This type of access should be reserved for unusual situations and granted only after careful deliberation by the ORP.

Non-public health uses of data: Release of data that are either directly or indirectly identifying to the public; to parties involved in civil, criminal, or administrative litigation; to non-public health agencies of the federal, state, or local government; or for commercial uses.

Overall responsible party (ORP): High-ranking official who accepts overall responsibility for implementing and enforcing data security standards. This official should have the authority to make decisions about program operations that might affect programs accessing or using the data, and should serve as contacts for public health professionals regarding security and confidentiality policies and practices. The ORP is responsible for protecting data as they are collected, stored, analyzed, and released and must certify annually that all security program requirements are being met. The state's security policy must indicate the ORP(s) by name.

Personnel controls: Staff member controls, such as training, separation of duties, and background checks, that are used as part of information security and management controls.

Personal identifier: Information that allows the identity of a person to be determined with a specified degree of certainty. This could be a single piece of information or several pieces of data which, when taken together, may be used to identify an individual. Therefore, when assembling or releasing analysis data sets, it is important to determine which fields, either alone or in combination, could be used to identify a person and which controls provide an acceptable level of security.

Personally identifiable information (PII): As defined by National Institute of Standards and Technology Special Publication 800-122, Guide to Protecting the Confidentiality of Personally Identifiable Information (PII), available at http://csrc.nist.gov/publications/: "Any information about an individual maintained by an agency, including (1) any information that can be used to distinguish or trace an individual's identity, such as name, social security number, date and place of birth, mother's maiden name, or biometric records; and (2) any other information that is linked or linkable to an individual, such as medical, educational, financial, and employment information."

Physical access controls: Physical barriers such as locked doors, sealed windows, password-protected keyboards, entry logs, guards, etc., used to help limit access to confidential information.

Public health surveillance: The ongoing, systematic collection, management, analysis, and interpretation of health-related data followed by their dissemination to those who need to know in order to: 1) monitor populations to detect unusual instances or patterns of disease, toxic exposure, or injury; 2) act to prevent or control these threats; and 3) intervene to promote and improve health. The term applies to both electronic and paper-based systems.

Public health data use (see also legitimate public health purpose): Includes the variety of ways public health data may be used to achieve public health goals/purposes. A principal public health data use at state and federal levels is for epidemiologic monitoring of trends in disease incidence and outcomes. This includes collection of data and evaluation of the collection system, as well as the dissemination of aggregate trends in incidence and prevalence by demographic, geographic, and behavioral risk characteristics to assist the formulation of public health policy and direct intervention programs. Public health data uses may also include data used to initiate or provide treatment and prevention services.

Records retention policy: A policy that stipulates how long paper and electronic records should be kept before they can be archived or destroyed.

Role-based access: Access to specific information or data granted on the basis of a person's job status or authority. This control mechanism protects data and system integrity by preventing access to unauthorized applications. Granting access based on roles within an organization, rather than by individual users, simplifies an organization's security policy and procedures and helps avoid granting need-to-know access to individuals.

Secure(d) area: Work space with physical access controls in which confidential data are kept and/or used with access granted only to authorized persons. The configuration of a secure(d) area depends on resource and other program considerations (e.g., availability of physical space, locks, file cabinets, walls, doors, and other barriers.)

Security: Protection of public health data and information systems to prevent unauthorized release of identifying information and accidental loss of data or damage to the systems. Security measures include measures to detect, document, and counter threats to data confidentiality or the integrity of data systems.

Syndemic: Synergist interaction of two or more conditions that contribute to an excess burden of disease in a population.

Virtual private network (VPN): Network of computers that uses encryption to scramble all data sent through the internet—making the network "virtually" private.

Appendix B.

Checklists for Assessment of Data Security and Confidentiality Protections

INITIAL ASSESSMENT

This checklist can be used to guide the initial assessment of a program's compliance with the Standards for Data Security and Confidentiality. This will be particularly useful for state and local public health programs that currently lack data security and confidentiality policies and procedures.

As indicated previously in this document, the initial assessment should be conducted by a team led by the ORP(s). The team should include:

- Program managers, directors, or equivalent leaders from participating programs
- Other representatives of participating programs
- Staff members with technical expertise in data security
- IT staff

The initial assessment should include the following steps:

- Identify key individuals and designate an ORP
- Review current security-related materials (e.g., written policies and procedures)
- Review relevant state and local laws that might affect data security and confidentiality policies
- Identify any policies or procedures that are either barriers to information sharing or sources of data security weaknesses
- Consult standard operating procedures (SOPs) from other programs that might be useful sources of ideas or suggestions for procedural changes
- Review any history of data security breaches or near-breaches, and associated lessons learned
- Assess physical security and define the secure area
- Assess electronic security protections and methods of data transfer and storage
- Assess factors related to security of information in the field, as appropriate
- Assess training needs

CONDUCTING AN INITIAL ASSESSMENT: STEPS AND GUIDING QUESTIONS

Identify key individuals and designate an ORP	Have key individuals, including program managers, directors, persons responsible for information and system security, and appropriate technical staff members, been identified?
	Has an ORP(s) with ultimate decision-making authority and responsibility for reconciling differences in policies and procedures across programs been identified?
Review current policies and gather resources	Have relevant policies, data-sharing agreements, and standard operating procedures been compiled and reviewed?
	Have relevant laws, rules, and regulations been considered?
Identify weaknesses and barriers	Have areas of weakness and specific topics that need additional clarification been identified?
	Have barriers to data sharing been identified?
	Have potential solutions to these barriers, including possible policy revisions, been noted?
Assess physical security and define the secure area	What is the work-space configuration?
	What is the path of public health data from collection and entry into the program's physical space through data entry and storage?
	What happens to case report forms received from providers? How are case report forms completed by health department staff handled? Is information obtained by phone or other electronic format? If so, how are hard copies or electronic media physically secured? Are electronic devices used, such as PDAs or laptops? If so, how are these physically secured?
	How is the area that houses identifiable data secured?
	Who has access to the physical space, who needs access, and for what purpose?
Assess electronic security, protections, and methods of data transfer and storage	Who or what roles need access to identifiable data? At what stage is their access required? Who needs access to electronic databases with identifiable data?
	Who needs access only to de-identified or analysis data sets?
	Who teleworks and what level of access do they need? Are electronic protections in place for remote access?
	Which individuals must take identifiable information in the field or outside of the secure physical area or health department? How is that information brought back into the office and what happens when it arrives?
	Does field work involve information on paper or electronic data on laptops or other storage devices?
	What electronic protections are in place during data transfer? Is encryption used? If so, when are data encrypted? Are data encrypted while at rest?
	Are data ever transported between locations across secured boundaries such as a secure data network (SDN), virtual private network, or Secure File Transfer Protocol (SFTP)?
Assess training needs	Do all programs involved have specific security and confidentiality training? How often is it conducted and who does it?
	What additional training will be required if policies are modified?
	Do other types of employees need to be trained (e.g. mail room staff, maintenance and cleaning staff, security staff, IT staff [in-house and contracted services])?
	How often are training materials updated?

Periodic Assessment Checklist

This checklist can be used to guide the periodic assessment of a program's compliance with the Standards for Data Security and Confidentiality.

For the answer to be "yes" to a question with multiple parts, all boxes must be checked. For each "No" response, provide additional information describing how the program intends to achieve compliance with that standard.

Name of Program being assessed

Name of person assessing the program

_____

_____

1.0 PROGRAM POLICIES AND RESPONSIBILITIES

STANDARD 1.1

In your program, how are staff members who are authorized to access HIV/VH/STD/TB information or data made aware of their data confidentiality and security responsibilities?

_____

_____

Are the following points addressed in your policies and agreements?

☐ Yes ☐ No	Are staff provided training on security policies and procedures and where to find resources?	
☐ Yes ☐ No	Does the program have written data security and confidentiality policies and procedures?	
☐ Yes ☐ No	Are written policies and procedures reviewed at least annually and revised as needed?	
☐ Yes ☐ No	Are data security policies readily accessible to all staff members who have access to confidential, individual-level data? Where are the policies located? _____	

STANDARD 1.2

☐ Yes ☐ No — In your program, is there a policy that assigns responsibilities and designates an ORP for the security of the data that is stored in various data systems?

☐ Yes ☐ No — Does the ORP have sufficient authority to make modifications to policies and procedures and ensure that the standards are met?

STANDARD 1.3

☐ Yes ☐ No — Does your program have a policy that defines the roles and access level for all persons with authorized access?

☐ Yes ☐ No — Does your program have a policy that describes which standard procedures or methods will be used when accessing HIV/VH/STD/TB information or other personally identifiable data?

STANDARD 1.4

☐ Yes ☐ No — Does the program have a written policy that describes the methods for ongoing review of technological aspects of security practices to ensure that data remain secure in light of evolving technologies?

STANDARD 1.5

☐ Yes ☐ No — Are written procedures in place to respond to breaches in procedures and breaches in confidentiality?
Where are those procedures stored? _____

☐ Yes ☐ No — Is the chain of communication and notification of appropriate individuals outlined in the data policy?

☐ Yes ☐ No — Are all breaches of protocol or procedures, regardless of whether personal information was released, investigated immediately to determine causes and implement remedies?

☐ Yes ☐ No — Are all breaches of confidentiality (i.e., a security infraction that results in the release of private information with or without harm to one or more persons) reported immediately to the ORP?

☐ Yes ☐ No — Do procedures include a mechanism for consulting with appropriate legal counsel to determine whether a breach warrants a report to law enforcement agencies?

☐ Yes ☐ No — If warranted, are law enforcement agencies contacted when a breach occurs?

☐ Yes ☐ No	Are staff trained on the program's definitions of breaches in procedures and breaches in confidentiality?
☐ Yes ☐ No	Are staff trained on ways to protect keys, use passwords, and codes that would allow access to confidential information or data?
☐ Yes ☐ No	Are staff trained on policies and procedures that describe how staff can protect program software from computer viruses and computer hardware from damage due to extreme heat or cold?
☐ Yes ☐ No	Have all persons authorized to access individual-level information been trained on the organization's information security policies and procedures?
☐ Yes ☐ No	Is every staff member, information technology (IT) staff member, and contractor who may need access to individual-level information or data required to attend security training annually?
☐ Yes ☐ No	Is the date of the training or test documented in the employee's personnel file?

STANDARD 1.7

☐ Yes ☐ No	Do all authorized staff members in your program sign a confidentiality agreement annually?
☐ Yes ☐ No	Do all newly hired staff members sign a confidentiality agreement before they are given authorization to access individual-level information and data?

STANDARD 1.8

☐ Yes ☐ No	Do policies state that staff are personally responsible for protecting their own computer workstation, laptop computer, or other devices associated with confidential public health information or data?
☐ Yes ☐ No	Are staff trained on ways to protect keys, use passwords, and codes that would allow access to confidential information or data?

STANDARD 1.9

☐ Yes ☐ No	Does your program certify annually that all program standards are met?

2.0 DATA COLLECTION AND USE

STANDARD 2.1

☐ Yes ☐ No   When public health data are shared or used, are the intended public health purposes and limits of how the data will be used adequately described?

STANDARD 2.2

☐ Yes ☐ No   When data are collected or shared, do they contain only the minimum information necessary to achieve the stated public health purpose?

STANDARD 2.3

☐ Yes ☐ No   Does your program explore alternatives to using identifiable data before sharing data, such as using anonymized or coded data?

What alternatives are currently in use in your program? _____

_____

STANDARD 2.4

☐ Yes ☐ No   Does your program have procedures in place to determine whether a proposed use of identifiable public health data constitutes research requiring IRB review?

3.0 DATA SHARING AND RELEASE

STANDARD 3.1

☐ Yes ☐ No   In your program, is access to HIV/VH/STD/TB information and data for any purposes unrelated to public health (e.g., litigation, discovery, or court order) only granted to the extent required by law?

What non-public health use of the data are required or allowed by law?

_____

STANDARD 3.2

◻ Yes ◻ No

When a proposed sharing of identifiable data is not covered by existing policies, does your program assess risks and benefits before making a decision to share data?

How are these risks assessed? _____

_____

STANDARD 3.3

◻ Yes ◻ No

When sharing personally identifiable HIV/VH/STD/TB information and/or data with other public health programs (i.e., those programs outside the primary program responsible for collecting and storing the data), is access to this information and/or data limited to those for whom the ORP:

◻ has weighed the benefits and risks of allowing access; and

◻ can verify that the level of security established is equivalent to these standards?

STANDARD 3.4

◻ Yes ◻ No

Is access to confidential HIV/VH/STD/TB information and data by personnel outside the HIV/VH/STD/TB programs:

◻ limited to those authorized based on an expressed and justifiable public health need?; and

◻ arranged in a manner that does not compromise or impede public health activities?; and

◻ carefully managed so as to not affect the public perception of confidentiality of the public health data collection activity and approved by the ORP?

◻ Yes ◻ No

Before allowing access to any HIV/VH/STD/TB data or information containing names for research or other purposes (e.g., for other than routine prevention program purposes), does your program require that the requester:

◻ demonstrate need for the names?; and

◻ obtain institutional review board (IRB) approval (if it has been determined to be necessary)?; and

◻ sign a confidentiality agreement?

STANDARD 3.5

☐ Yes ☐ No Does your program have written procedures to review data releases that are not covered under the standing data release policy?

If not, does your program have unwritten policy to review data releases that are not covered under the standing data release policy?

☐ Yes ☐ No

Describe briefly those procedures or policies: _____

_____

STANDARD 3.6

☐ Yes ☐ No Does your program routinely distribute nonidentifiable summary data to stakeholders?

STANDARD 3.7

☐ Yes ☐ No Does your program assess data for quality before disseminated?

STANDARD 3.8

☐ Yes ☐ No Does the program have a data-release policy that defines access to, and use of, individual-level information?

☐ Yes ☐ No Does the data-release policy incorporate provisions to protect against public access to raw data or data tables that include small denominator populations that could be indirectly identifying information?

4.0 PHYSICAL SECURITY

Are workspaces and paper copies for persons working with confidential, individual-level information located within a secure, locked area?

☐ Yes ☐ No

- ☐ Are sensitive documents stored in cabinets?
- ☐ Are the cabinets locked?
- ☐ Are cabinets located in an area to which there is no access by unauthorized employees?
- ☐ Are cabinets located in an area to which there is no public access?

☐ Yes ☐ No

Do program staff members shred documents containing confidential information with a cross-cutting shredder before disposing of them?

☐ Yes ☐ No

Does your program have a written policy that outlines procedures for handling paper documents which could contain confidential information that are mailed to, or from, the program?

☐ Yes ☐ No

Do staff members in your program ensure that the amount and sensitivity of information contained in any piece of correspondence remains minimal?

☐ Yes ☐ No

Is access to all secured areas where confidential, individual-level HIV/VH/STD/TB information and data are stored limited to persons who are authorized within policies and procedures (this includes access by cleaning or maintenance staff)?

☐ Yes ☐ No	Do policies include procedures for securing documents containing PII when they cannot be returned to a secure work site by the close of business?
☐ Yes ☐ No	Do policies outline specific reasons, permissions and physical security procedures for using, transporting and protecting documents containing PII in a vehicle or personal residence?
☐ Yes ☐ No	If no such procedure exists, is approval obtained from the program manager?

STANDARD 4.6

☐ Yes ☐ No	When identifying information is taken from secured areas and included in on-line lists or supporting notes, in either electronic or hard-copy format: ☐ is it assured that the documents contain only the minimum amount of information necessary for completing a given task?, and ☐ is the information encrypted?, and ☐ is it coded to disguise information that could be easily associated with individuals?
☐ Yes ☐ No	Do staff members in your program ensure that terms easily associated with HIV/VH/STD/TB do not appear anywhere in the context of data transmissions, including sender and recipient addresses and labels?

5.0 ELECTRONIC DATA SECURITY

STANDARD 5.1

☐ Yes ☐ No	In your program, are HIV/VH/STD/TB analysis data sets stored securely using protective software (i.e., software that controls the storage, removal, and use of the data)?
☐ Yes ☐ No	Are personal identifiers removed from HIV/VH/STD/TB analysis data sets whenever possible?

In your program, do transfers of HIV/VH/STD/TB data and information and methods for data collection:

☐ Yes ☐ No

- ☐ have the approval of the ORP?, and
- ☐ incorporate the use of access controls?, and
- ☐ encrypt individual-level information and data before electronic transfer?

☐ Yes ☐ No — When possible, are databases and files with individual-level data encrypted when not in use?

☐ Yes ☐ No — Does your program have a policy that outlines procedures for handling electronic information and data (including, but not limited to, e-mail and fax transmissions) which may contain confidential information that are sent electronically to or from the program?

When individual-level HIV/VH/STD/TB information or data are electronically transmitted and the transmission does not incorporate the use of an encryption package meeting the encryption standards of the National Institute of Standards and Technology and approved by the ORP, are the following conditions met?

☐ Yes ☐ No

- ☐ The transmission does not contain identifying information.
- ☐ Terms easily associated with HIV/VH/STD/TB do not appear anywhere in the context of the transmission, including the sender and recipient address and label.

For all laptop computers and other portable devices (e.g., personal digital assistants [PDAs], other handheld devices, and tablet personal computers [tablet PCs]), which receive or store HIV/VH/STD/TB information or data with personal identifiers, are all the following steps taken to ensure the security of the data?

- [ ] Yes - [ ] No

☐ The devices have encryption software that meets federal standards.

☐ Program information with identifiers is encrypted and stored on an external storage device or on the laptop's removable hard drive.

☐ External storage devices or hard drives containing the information are separated from the laptop and held securely when not in use.

☐ The decryption key is kept some place other than on the device.

- [ ] Yes - [ ] No

Do the methods employed for sanitizing a storage device ensure that the information cannot be retrieved using "undelete" or other data retrieval software?

- [ ] Yes - [ ] No

Does the program have policies or procedures to ensure that all removable or external storage devices containing HIV/VH/STD/TB information or data that contain personal identifiers:

☐ include only the minimum amount of information necessary to accomplish assigned tasks as determined by the program manager, and

☐ are encrypted or stored under lock and key when not in use, and

☐ are sanitized immediately after a given task (excludes devices used for backups)?

Where are these policies or procedures stored? _____

- [ ] Yes - [ ] No

Are hard drives that contain identifying information sanitized or destroyed before the computers are labeled as excess or surplus, reassigned to nonprogram staff members, or sent off site for repair?

- [ ] Yes - [ ] No

Does your program have policies for handling incoming and outgoing facsimile transmissions to minimize risk of inadvertent disclosure of PII?

Appendix C.

Data Sharing Scenario

The following scenario is an example of data sharing between HIV and STD programs. In this scenario, a new case patient with HIV infection is identified through HIV surveillance and is offered partner services by the STD program. This scenario will not apply to all programs, but rather highlights one method for data sharing.

State and local health departments are notified of previously unknown patients with HIV infection by public or private laboratories that submit electronic or hard-copy laboratory and/or case reports indicative of HIV infection. The reports may be sent to a state health department, where HIV and STD staff may assign the newly identified patient to a local health department for partner services. Sometimes a laboratory will send the report directly to a local health department, and the staff there may immediately begin the process of offering partner services.

This example illustrates the information flow when a state health department receives an electronic laboratory report of HIV infection and shares that information with the local health department staff for partner services.

At the Home State Health Department, the STD program conducts partner services for both HIV and STD. However, the HIV surveillance unit operates separately from the STD program, thus requiring data sharing between programs. As an initial step, Jim, the HIV surveillance coordinator at the Home State Health Department, receives an electronic laboratory report for what appears to be a new case patient with HIV infection. He conducts a search through eHARS and confirms that this patient has not been previously reported.

When Jim enters the HIV case report information into eHARS, he notes that there is incomplete or missing information on the laboratory report. Referring to the Home State Data Sharing Plan, Jim provides the minimal information that he has on this case to the State Health Department STD program which forwards it to the Field Supervisor in the STD program at the Small City Health Department which is in the jurisdiction in which the patient resides. Jim sends a hard copy of the HIV case report form to the STD program with the patient's name, date of birth, gender, home address and telephone number, and current HIV test information. He also includes a request to obtain missing demographic, risk factor, HIV testing, and HIV treatment information from the patient during the partner services investigation.

The state health department HIV surveillance unit provided enough information to initiate a field record which is then assigned to a team of Disease Intervention Specialists (DISs). Jane, a DIS in the local health department's STD program, receives the HIV field record from her First-Line Supervisor (FLS) and conducts a record search to determine whether the patient has been previously notified of their HIV status, received Partner Services, or been reported to the health department for any other STDs. Jane determines that this individual has not had any of these encounters with the health department. Jane goes to the field to locate, notify, and interview the client. Jane locates and interviews the client and provides counseling and Partner Services. Jane makes sure to document any missing demographic and risk information to include in the case records and to share the missing information with HIV surveillance.

During the investigation, Jane also offers the client STD testing and referral for medical management of HIV infection, which typically includes TB screening and may include Hepatitis B vaccination or Hepatitis C screening. Upon returning to the local health department, Jane completes the case documentation and enters the data into the electronic STD data management and reporting system. Jane shares the results of the field investigation with the STD Field Supervisor and provides documentation of the missing HIV information to the HIV surveillance unit, according to instructions in the Home State Health Department's Data Sharing Plan.

The following flow diagram outlines the above scenario.

HIV/AIDS PARTNER SERVICES (PS) DATA
FLOW CHART

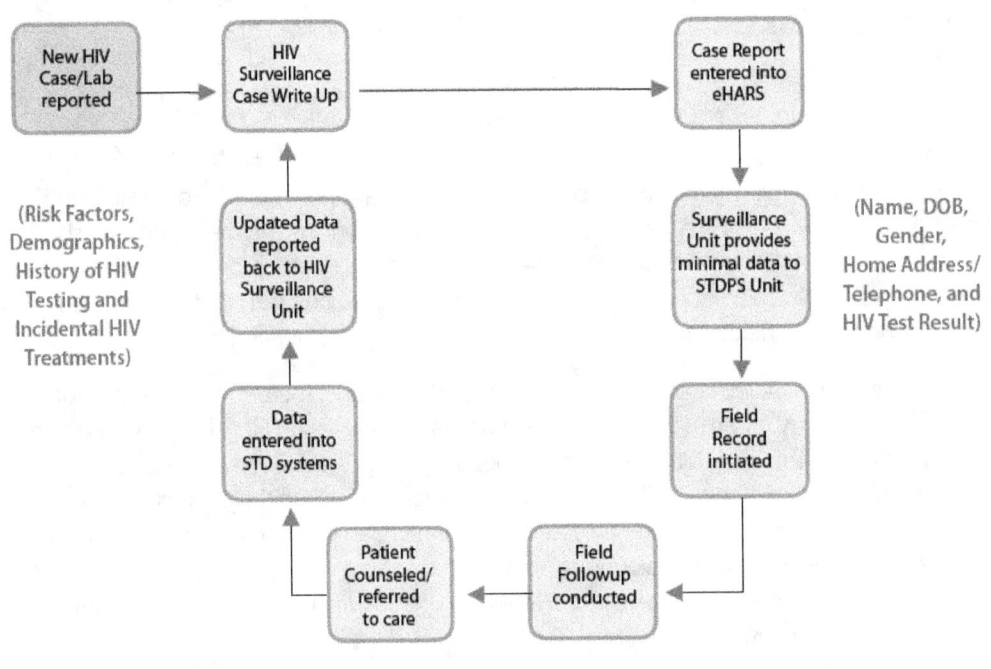

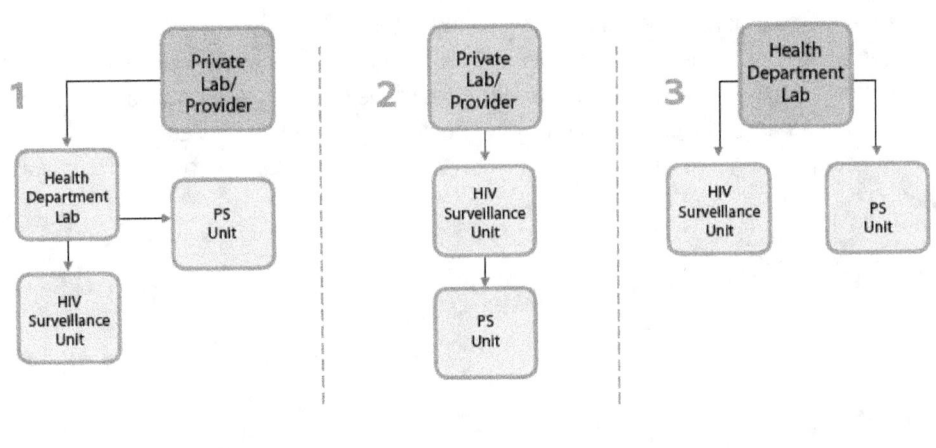

Appendix D.

Sample Certification Statement

CERTIFICATION OF COMPLIANCE
WITH THE "SECURITY AND CONFIDENTIALITY STANDARDS FOR PUBLIC HEALTH DATA AND DESIGNATION OF OVERALL RESPONSIBLE PARTY (ORP)"

By signing and submitting this form, we certify our compliance with "NCHHSTP Security and Confidentiality Guidelines." We acknowledge that all standards included in the NCHHSTP Security and Confidentiality Guidelines have been implemented unless otherwise justified in an attachment to this statement. We agree to apply the standards to all local/state staff and contractors funded through NCHHSTP that have access to or maintain confidential public health data. We ensure all sites where applicable public health data are maintained are informed about the standards. Documentation of required local data policies and procedures is on file with the ORP and available upon request.

Name(s), occupation, and organizational affiliation of the proposed ORP.

NAME	TITLE	AFFILIATION

Applicant/Grantee Name

Grant/Cooperative Agreement Number

Signature: Principle Investigator

Signature: Authorized Business Official

Date

Date

Appendix E.

Suggested Outline for a Policy on Data Confidentiality, Security, Sharing, and Use

The following is an outline of suggested components of a policy on data confidentiality, security, sharing and use that can be adapted to local needs.

- Scope
  - » Relevant data
  - » Purpose of the data collection(s)
  - » Terms of use and data sharing
  - » Ten guiding principles for data security, confidentiality, sharing, and use
  - » Reference to each of the standards for data security, confidentiality, sharing and use
- Access and roles
  - » Level of access to confidential surveillance data by position (including staff who use the data daily as well as IT/data management staff)
  - » Roles of persons who have/need access to data
- Overall responsible party (ORP)
- Data release
  - » Rules governing release of individual and aggregate data (with reference to a separate data release policy document, as indicated)
  - » Methods by which information will be disseminated and shared (including circumstances requiring a data-release agreement)
- Data-sharing agreements/plans
  - » Procedures for implementing data-sharing agreements/plans, as indicated
  - » IRB procedures, if IRB approval required
- Routine communications with confidential, identifiable data
  - » Procedures for communications requiring the sharing of confidential, identifiable data with other project areas, both intra- and interstate and providers, laboratories, and other internal and external entities
- Physical data security
  - » Procedures to ensure a secure physical environment (e.g., access to rooms, security screens, backup storage, file cabinets, storage of hard copies, use of shipping companies, opening of mail, and removal of information from secure areas)

- Electronic data security

  » Procedures to ensure a secure electronic environment (e.g., transfer and storage of electronic data, data backups, use of different media devices [PDAs, tablets, laptops, and thumb drives], and encryption requirements)

- Transmission of data

  » Procedures on transmission of data via physical mail, fax, e-mail, and other emerging electronic/wireless technologies

- Investigation of suspected breaches

  » Processes, tools, and forms to investigate and document suspected breaches of protocol and/or confidentiality

  » Chain of information/action/response

- Training

  » Requirements for annual, standard training on data security confidentiality policies and procedures, including a review of the written documents

  » Requirements for documentation of training

- Nondisclosure or confidentiality agreements

- Glossary

Appendix F.

Guidelines for the Use of Facsimile Machines*

Although facsimile (fax) equipment and software can enhance the quality of health care by facilitating rapid transmission of health information, this same mode of transmission opens up the possibility that information will be misdirected or intercepted by persons for whom access is not intended or authorized. In recent years, numerous reports have described events wherein patient health records were inadvertently faxed to a wrong location (e.g., bank or retail store) rather than the intended recipient. The following recommendations will help minimize the risks associated with use of facsimile machines.

- Establish fax policies and procedures based on federal guidelines, state laws and regulations, and consultation with legal counsel, as needed.

- Take reasonable steps to ensure that the fax transmission is sent to the intended destination. As possible, pre-program and periodically audit and test destination numbers to eliminate errors in transmission from misdialing and outdated fax numbers. Periodically, remind frequent recipients of PII to notify the program of any changes in fax number. Train staff to double check the recipient's fax number before pressing the 'send' key.

- Provide education and training to staff on the program's fax policies and procedures. This includes educating private providers and laboratories that report information to public health programs. Take reasonable operational safeguards to alert staff of faxing procedures. For example, affix brightly colored stickers to fax machines reminding staff of key fax policies (e.g., need for a cover sheet; verification of recipient's fax number; and procedures to implement if an incoming fax has been received in error).

- Require all fax communications be sent with a cover sheet that includes name and contact information of the sender and the recipient, confidentiality disclaimer statement, and instructions on what to do if the document is received in error (see Sample Confidentiality Disclaimer below).

- If a fax transmission fails to reach the recipient, check the internal logging system of the fax machine to obtain the number to which the transmission was sent. If the sender becomes aware that a fax was misdirected, contact the receiver and ask that the material be returned or destroyed. Investigate misdirected faxes as a risk management occurrence or security incident, inform the ORP, and log the incident for remediation/mitigation.

- Locate fax machines in secure areas.

- Ensure that data security policies include procedures for maintaining and disposing of paper fax transmissions.

Sample Confidentiality Disclaimer

The documents accompanying this fax transmission contain health information that is legally privileged. This information is intended only for the use of the individual or entity named above. The authorized recipient of this information is prohibited from disclosing this information to any other party unless required to do so by law or regulation and is required to destroy the information after its stated need has been fulfilled. If you are not the intended recipient, you are hereby notified that any disclosure, copying, distribution, or action taken in reliance on the contents of these documents is strictly prohibited. If you have received this information in error, please notify the sender immediately and arrange for the return or destruction of these documents.

Based on "Facsimile Transmission of Health Information"
http://library.ahima.org/xpedio/groups/public/documents/ahima/bok1_031811.hcsp?dDocName=bok1_031811

Appendix G.

Ensuring Data Security in Nontraditional Work Settings

Electronic Data Security

The following restrictions must be followed when dealing with personally identifiable information (PII) in a telework environment.

- The media on the device being used to access PII must be fully encrypted; encryption of individual files is not adequate.

- Personal computers or personal electronic media should not be used for data storage. Data-storage devices must be issued by the agency. On an agency-issued device, internet service provider (ISP) or personal network equipment may be used for internet connectivity.

- Agency-issued computers must be configured to prevent installation of software by persons other than agency IT staff.

- The agency must have properly configured firewalls installed on computers to be used outside of the agency's protective boundaries.

- PII should never reside on a device that is ever connected to the internet either directly or indirectly outside the agency firewall.

- PII may be analyzed if technology is used to access and analyze remotely with only displays of data and results being shown on the device. Citrix applications are an example of this technology.

Telework

Teleworking is a complex issue, particularly because most of the work performed by surveillance and field staff involves patient identifiers or potential identifiers. Whenever possible, work with surveillance data should be performed at the worksite, with recommended physical, electronic, and procedural protections. Even though IT staff may make it possible to have the same access at home that is available in the office, that does not mean that the access or home workplace is just as secure.

Nonetheless, current workplace trends are moving strongly toward teleworking, even for individuals working with PII. Therefore, programs should coordinate with IT and their own staff to ensure that home access meets the same confidentiality and security protections as the office work space. The work environment of the teleworker should be subject to an audit to verify minimum physical security protections.

Recommended characteristics of a telework location include:

- Limited access (e.g., a locking door) in a private area. In a home, this means a dedicated room with no access by unauthorized persons. The ability to observe PII on device displays must be restricted to only the teleworker.

- No hard-copy storage of client-identified data. If hard copies of any documents must be stored in a telework location, they should be stored in double-locked file cabinets, large and heavy enough to render them immobile. Hard copies of documents containing PII must be shredded using a cross-cut shredder and should never to be left in an unsecured area.

- The work space must be configured to allow confidential conversations.

  » PII stored and transmitted via a computer with encryption software at least equal to the currently accepted level of encryption used in the regular workplace

  » If the computer is connected to the internet with Wi-Fi, access to the Wi-Fi connection must be secure.

Field/Clinic work

Many public health workers handle PII in the field while pursuing public health activities. Traditionally, most of that data has been in hard copy, but the evolving technology of PDAs, electronic tablets, and notebook computers is driving many programs away from traditional paper data to e-data stored on portable devices. Programs must therefore plan for migration from paper-oriented to electronic systems that meet established and evolving electronic and procedural security standards. Forward-looking confidentiality and security protocols should include provisions for phones, PDAs, tablets, and workbooks that take client-identified data to the field and allow for real-time updates, reporting, and data entry from field sites as well as by medical staff in examination rooms. These protocols should also provide accountability measures to ensure that staff members employ this secured, confidential data in appropriate locations while in the field. Programs may review Guidelines on Cell Phone and PDA Security, National Institute of Standards and Technology Special Publication 800-124, available at http://csrc.nist.gov/publications/, when developing policies.

Remote work

In the case of emergency or outbreak responses, staff may be detailed to work sites that have not been prepared to meet data security standards. The host area and detailed staff should ensure that the work site is made as secure as reasonably possible in terms of physical, electronic, and procedural security.

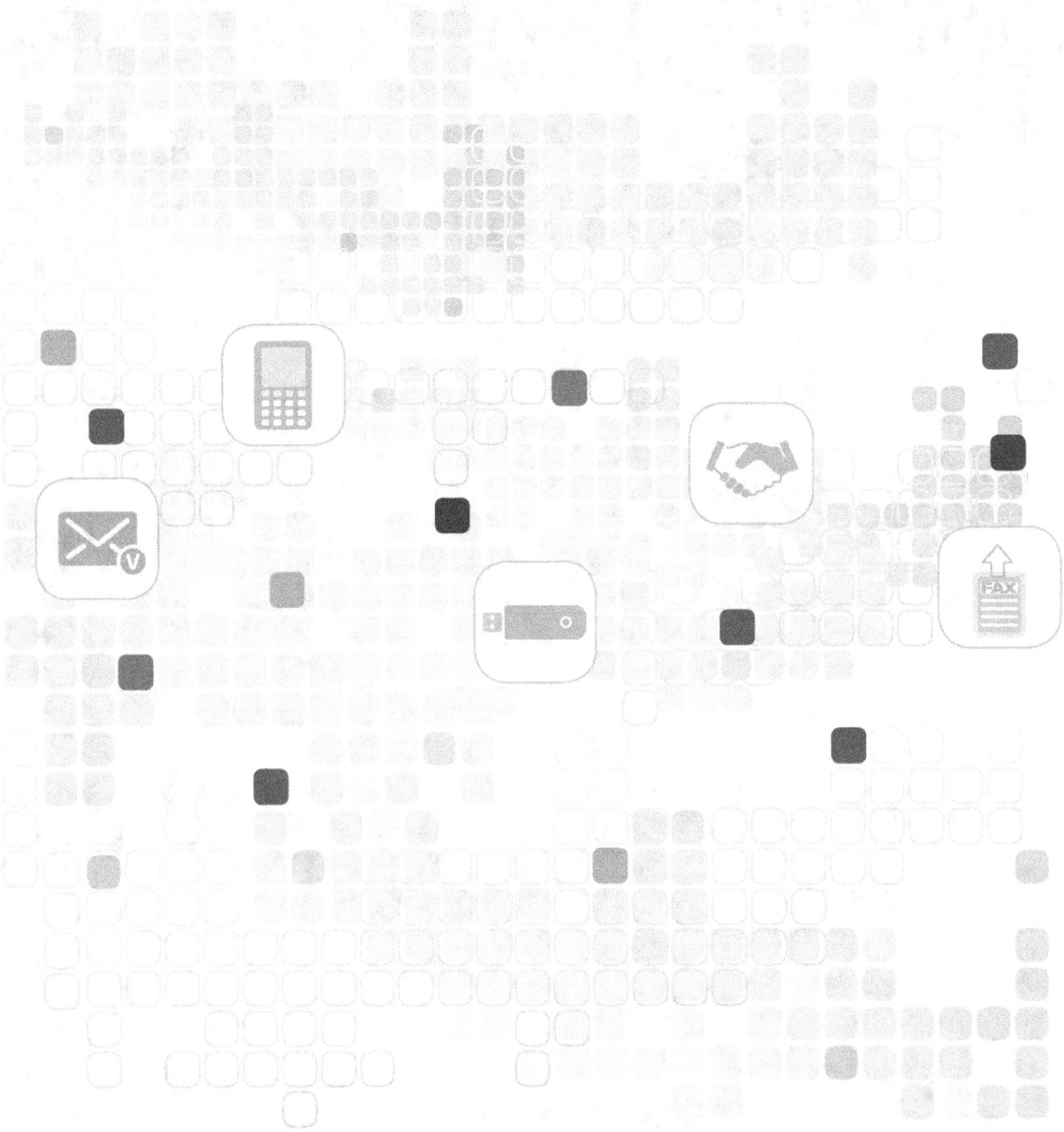

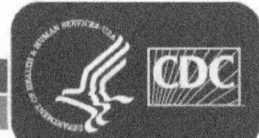